THE CELESTIAL STEMS

Provides a definitive explanation of what exactly the Celestial Stems are, and how to apply the knowledge in daily acupuncture practice.

By the same author
ACUPUNCTURE ATLAS AND REFERENCE BOOK
PRINCIPLES AND PRACTICE OF MOXIBUSTION
(with Roger Newman Turner)
THE SECONDARY VESSELS OF ACUPUNCTURE

THE CELESTIAL STEMS

by

Royston Low
Ph.D., N.D., D.O., M.B.N.O.A., F.B.Ac.A., Dr.Ac.

THORSONS PUBLISHERS LIMITED
Wellingborough, Northamptonshire

THORSONS PUBLIHERS INC.
New York

First published 1985

British Library Cataloguing in Publication Data

Low, Royston
The celestial stems.
1. Acupuncture
I. Title
615.8'92 RM184

ISBN 0-7225-0788-7

Printed and bound in Great Britain

To
Eunice, Ian and Christopher,
and to all those unseen helpers
who provide the most timely
though unexpected inspiration.

CONTENTS

ACKNOWLEDGEMENTS

For a subject such as this the sources have to be many and varied. I have drawn heavily upon the works of Joseph Needham, Chaumfrault and Van Nghi, Manfred Porkert, and Henry Lu. Each provided a part of the puzzle and although at times inevitable contradictions crept in, eventually a glimmer of light appeared and things started to fall into place.

The quotations from the Nei Ching are all from Henry Lu's translation, and I have also utilized his method of working out the points detailed in Chapter 5 — 'The Daily Cycle'.

I would like to express my thanks to Shyam Singha for certain insights into basic Chinese philosophy and its relationship to the Tridosha which he gave in lectures to the Acupuncture Research Association as long ago as 1962.

INTRODUCTION

Western critics of traditional Chinese acupuncture claim that it is too esoteric in its approach — that the concepts of Ch'i energy, of Yin and Yang, of the Five Transformations (or Five Elements) are basically unscientific, unproven and totally unnecessary, and serve only to obscure the basic simplicity. The fact that 'Western' acupuncturists get very limited results they ascribe to limitations of acupuncture itself rather than to their own ignorance of the very elements of the art.

At the extreme other end of the spectrum are those Traditionalists who maintain that it is impossible to be a Master of Acupuncture without a complete knowledge of the 'Celestial Stems' and the 'Terrestrial Branches', and of how to apply this in practice.

According to Needham, Chapters 66 to 71 in the *Su Wen*, which are the chapters dealing with this approach, are heavily suspect, as they do not appear earlier than editions presented by Wang Ping in AD 762.

It is possible that it is based on ideas first put forward by divisors such as Ching Fang (45 BC) and incorporated into the *I Ching* during the Hun period, but by the twelfth century it had been fully incorporated into the medical classics of the time.

Be that as it may, like so many other things in life it appears as if all progress is truly a spiral, and the circle is once more swinging around to complete itself on a slightly higher level, with a growing awareness that some of the old concepts had much truth in them

— a truth which does not conflict with modern inductive reasoning but rather complements and enhances it.

So what are the 'Celestial Stems'? They are based on the realization that the affairs of Man are affected by cosmic and planetary influences on all levels of being, from the macrocosmic to the microscopic, and they attempt to describe just what those prevailing influences are, at any given moment, and how the energies inherent in man will react to them.

Only within the last few decades has the truth of these ancient ideas been forced upon us, and the more we learn about the workings of the human body the more we realize that the individual is affected both mentally and physically by climatic and meteorological conditions beyond his control, and that the body possesses its own specific daily, monthly and yearly cycles.

The daily rhythms are well-known as the circadian cycles, the body's 'biological clock'. Traditional acupuncture speaks of the ebb and flow of Yin and Yang — of Yang being most active in the morning to reach its maximum at noon, with a slow change into Yin until Yin climaxes at midnight to change slowly back into Yang with the advent of the new day. It speaks also of the well-known 24-hour cycle of energy, with the meridial energy awakening in the lungs at 3 a.m. and progressing through the twelve meridians in a regular order through the day:

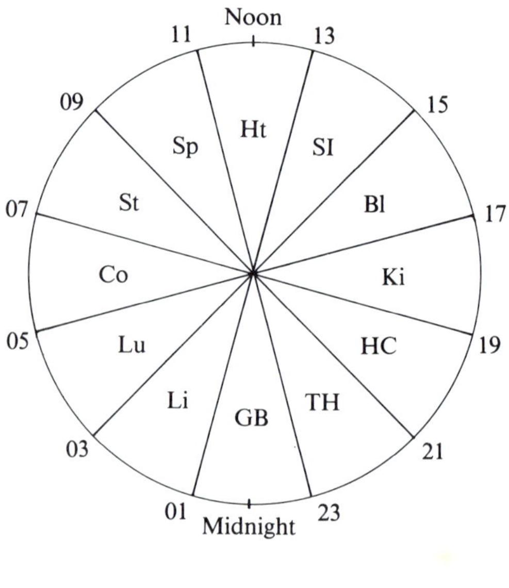

Modern research has drawn the parallel to this in the discovery that both hormones and the activity of the auto-immune system follow a similar pattern. Corticosterone and plasma ACTH also peak at noon, fall off during the afternoon to a minimum at midnight, and then slowly increase again. Many other hormones concerned with tissue growth and regeneration behave in the same way, as do the cyclic nucleotides. The phenomenon of 'jet-lag', when our circadian rhythms are upset, is too well-known to need description.

That our bodies could be affected by the position of the moon was a proposition long regarded as pure superstition by the world of 'scientific' medicine. Agreed that the word 'lunacy' was always used to describe mental aberration, but that it could be founded to some extent on fact was disregarded. But the ancient worship of Isis, the moon or mother goddess, was not without some justification — the fact that a woman's menstrual cycle is under lunar domination is evident to all, and the tides which affect the seas also affect the life-cycles of its inhabitants.

The ancient Chinese observations of the effects of the moon in this respect were acute, as observed by Needham (*Science and Civilisation in China*, Vol. 3) in his quotation from Yen Su's *Hai C'hao Tu Lun* (*circa* 1030):

> The original forces breathe in and out, and the sky following the forces expands and contracts, while the tide going and coming in the seas follows the sky and flows and ebbs. Since the sun is the mother of the double Yang, and Yin is born of Yang, the tide is subject to the sun; and since the moon is the essence of the Yin, and water is Yin, the tide follows the motions of the moon. For this reason, following the sun and responding to the moon, copying the motions of the Yin and yet subject to the Yang, the tide is at its highest at new and full moon, contracts as the moon waxes or wanes, is at its lowest at the first and last quarter, and grows just before full and new moon. That is the reason why there are large and small tides.

The existence of monthly (circatrigintan) rhythms is being verified more and more, as are slightly broader, more seasonal variations, tending to bear out the so-called 5-Phase or 5-Element relationships, i.e., the activity of the liver in spring, the heart in summer, the spleen in long summer, the lungs in autumn, and the kidneys in winter. The variations in pulse quality associated with seasonal changes are also now being verified objectively.

Even more interesting are the effects of the individual biorhythms — the fact that every person has their own particular cycles:

> 23 day physical, of the cells controlling the muscular and physical system.
> 28 day emotional, of the cells controlling the nervous system.
> 33 day intellectual, of the cells controlling the brain.

These are activated from the moment of birth, and manifest as a sine-wave with plus and minus phases of activity.

The effects of any of the aforementioned factors are therefore modified by the state of the individual's own rhythms at any particular time, and the effect of, and response to, treatment will also vary correspondingly.

This will explain, to the discerning practitioner, why the effects from his treatment will vary from day to day and from patient to patient, and why patients respond more readily on some days than on others — also why Dai Qui is obtained more quickly on certain points at certain times. All experienced practitioners will have noticed this — the explanation lies in the present subject of discussion.

As will be described in the following chapters, there are really several aspects to this approach — the first is the overall dominant influence of the year itself within the Chinese 60-year cycle; then there is the seasonal influence within the year, and finally there is the influence of the specific day and time of day upon the individual.

The overall cosmic influences are the Celestial Stems. There are ten of them, and as they are the influences of Heaven upon Earth they are Yang by nature. The 'guest' energies with which they interact are called the Terrestrial Branches — they number twelve, and are Yin by nature.

On the so-called Great Cycle the stems and branches are both years, with reaction between the dominant aspect of the greater 60-year cycle and the smaller 10-year one upon the specific year, and give the overall 'flavour' of the year itself.

On the 'lesser' cycle the stems are the years (in the 10-year cycle) and the branches are the months.

In the monthly cycle, the stems are the months (seasons) and the branches are the days.

In the daily cycle, the stems are the days and the branches are the twelve divisions of the 24 hours, and the meridians appertaining thereto.

To add confusion to understanding, regardless of the cycle under consideration, the names of the Ten Celestial Stems and the Twelve Terrestrial Branches remain constant. (I have given the names in the Wade-Giles Romanization; where the Pinyin is different I have put it in brackets):

Stems	
Chia (Jia)	甲
Yee (Yi)	乙
Ping (Bing)	丙
Ding	丁
Wu	戊
Ji	己
Geng	庚
Hsin (Xin)	辛
Ren	壬
Gui	癸

Branches	
Tzu (Zi)	子
Chou	丑
Yin	寅
Mao	卯
Chen	辰
Si	巳
Wu	午
Wei	未
Shen	申
Yu	酉
Shu (Xu)	戌
Hai	亥

Table 1.

For an understanding of this subject one has to realize that all science and philosophy has its birth in the attempt of primitive man to come to terms with the universe as he saw it. From the earliest days his life was governed by forces beyond his control and comprehension, and by attempting to describe and understand those forces he felt that he could somehow bring them more under his control and thus possibly alleviate his lot.

In attempting to understand them, he resorted to the erection of philosophical concepts which were, naturally, limited by the environment and ecology in which he existed. In all parts of the world he looked at the stars, and in particular the sun and the moon, and wondered. The stars he could not comprehend — those little twinkling motes above his head — but the sun and the moon

— they were powerful; by their appearance and disappearance they heralded the warmth and the cold, the light and the dark, the abundance or lack of food both animal and vegetable upon which his survival depended. Such powerful beings needed to be propitiated, and they became gods to whom regular sacrifices had to be offered to secure their favour.

But whilst, in the West, primitive man huddled in his caves and devised elaborate ceremonies of propitiation, in the East an older race was looking, wondering and pondering. Their savants were absorbed by the eternal interplay of heat and cold, light and dark, inter- and re-action, and evolved the hypothesis that all life was a balance of two opposing forces, which they termed Yin and Yang.

Slowly a concept began to emerge. The beginning was unknowable — it was the Dao, the point within a circle which had no beginning and no end. It was all, it was nothing, the Alpha and the Omega; it existed of and from itself and yet, because it was unmanifest, its ability for action remained as a pure potential. That potential could only be realized by activity, the ability to change, and the 'Great Principle of Change' was the Tai I. The One became Two, and with the formation of Two the facility for interaction was produced, so that Two could become Three and matter could begin to appear.

The first element to form was Water (equated with hydrogen), then came the formation of Fire as its opposite. From compression of the Fire energy came the formation of Wood (activity) and from this activity came form and Metal. From Metal (the element which cools Fire) came Earth, and Earth produced 'the myrial beings, who carry Yin on their backs and embrace Yang'.

The lighter elements, tending upwards, produced Heaven and were Yang; the heavier, sinking to and producing Earth, were Yin, and Man was the result of the interplay of these two forces, carrying within himself the seeds of light and dark, of good and evil, of selfishness and selflessness — of Yin and Yang — the microcosm in the macrocosm.

Man also possessed the ability to look both inwards and outwards. Looking inwards he discovered the seeds of wonder and the existence of the Dao within himself; looking outwards, he perceived the starry firmament and the manifestation of the Dao through the whole of the universe. And he was content to know that he and the Dao were one.

1.
PHILOSOPHICAL BACKGROUND

'The square pertains to Earth, the circle belongs to Heaven, Heaven being round and the Earth square.'*

— Chou Pei Suan Ching

'Heaven corresponds to the base of a right-angled triangle, Earth to the height, Man to the hypotenuse, and Things to the diameter of a circle inscribed in the triangle.'

— Tsu I-Chi in preface to *Su Yuan Yü Chien*

To fully comprehend the metaphysics involved one has to approach from the basis of symbolism. The use of symbols is the only way in which our minds, limited by the information provided by our five senses, can attempt to define and understand that which is beyond and behind the material universe. All study of metaphysics invariably ends up by considering the theological, and it is interesting to reflect that formalized religion always appears to have followed one of two paths, the 'inductive' and the 'deductive'.

Many primitive religions start off as a worship of individual spirits thought to be inherent in all the myriad aspects of nature — a primitive pantheism in which every rock, tree, stream or mountain had its own guardian angel or demon, naiad or dryad,

*Three, the number of Heaven and the nearest approximation to π was a male or Yang number, whilst four, the number of Earth, was a female or Yin.

to be appeased or propitiated. With increasing sophistication gradually came the concepts of higher deities — the powers behind the scenes — until eventually the one supreme god emerged — Father of all — Zeus, Jupiter, Jehovah, Odin, Quetzalcoatl — his name is legion.

The other approach is the exact opposite in which the primary concept is, as I have said in the Introduction, a feeling that the beginning of all was unknowable, existing on a plane far removed from the physical through which it manifests itself. It was to be revered or respected, in that it was the higher aspect of Man himself, who was part of it, yet it was not to be bowed down to or propitiated. Teleology held true for both concepts, yet the first was far more anthropomorphic, with God created in Man's own image, whilst the second was purely philosophical and far more wide-ranging in its implications. But the part cannot comprehend the whole, and to bring the incomprehensible down to a level where man could begin to reach some form of rapport the greater whole had to be broken down into smaller parts, which man could — just — begin to grasp hold of and imagine. These smaller parts — the various attributes of deity — in turn were projected as stylized symbols through which the deity could be approached, and thus were derived the various multiple gods of the Ancient Egyptians and the Hindu pantheons, frequently bearing the heads of those animals thought to epitomize their specific characteristics.

The difference between these religions and the former, however, is that their followers are aware that their 'gods' are symbols, and merely artefacts erected by the limited human brain to enable it to 'tune-in' to the invisible essence behind the illusory world of the five senses. On the lowest level one is in the ground-floor with priestly ritual prevailing, but the higher one ascends so one reaches into the realms of mysticism and non-attachment to the physical by which means alone can true understanding be obtained.

As has been pointed out by that great savant C. G. Jung, it is amazing how all minds, regardless of their environmental or ethnic milieu, seem to employ the same symbols for the same concepts. Thus he derived the theory of the archetypical subconscious. And, again as mentioned in the Introduction, the almost universally accepted symbol for the original Absolute, from which all derived, was the Point, infinitesimally small, existing in its own space and time, yet bearing within itself the seeds of the whole cosmos. Yet the Point, on its own, was impotent. It could do, or be, nothing unless there was some opposite with which it could interact — and thus the One, manifesting itself as its own opposite reflection, became Two, and initiated the birth of Yin and Yang — Light and Dark, Ormazd and Ahriman. Yet still the Two were incomplete — they existed of, and from, themselves, yet in themselves were nothing, for of what use were Light and Dark if there was nothing upon which they could shine. And so the Two came together and the Two became Three, and the creation of Matter began.

•	Point
• •	Male and Female
• • •	Matter

Nearly all religions bear witness to this subconscious stylization — Isis and Osiris with the infant Horus, the Holy Trinity of Father, Son and Holy Ghost, or the Hindu Brahma, Vishnu and Siva (the two latter symbolizing the creative and annihilative powers of the Deity).

An extension of this idea again begins with the 'point' ● , and the point issues from itself the primal force (the 'Word' of the Scriptures) which is symbolized by the straight line ' | '. This is the male principle. But the force is meaningless unless there is a matrix in which it can embody itself — the 'Womb of Night', the 'Primeval Chaos' — pictured as a circle O , the female principle. And so we have the two oldest symbols in the world, the Lingam and the Yoni, the male and female — | O . Yet still it is meaningless — the principles are united — ⦶ , but the Two have still to become Three — ⊕ , and matter is born. But the child is still in the womb — matter is still locked in its spiritual matrix and has to stand free — + . Since time immemorial, long before its adoption by Christianity, the cross in one or other of its forms has been utilized as the symbol for matter (ponder on the meaning of the Crux Ansata!) and matter alone exists in the four dimensions of Space and Time — matter is 'Four Square' □. So the square is also a symbol for matter, and in Chinese philosophy the circle has always stood for spirit and the square for the material.

• | ○ ⦶ ⊕ + □

An interesting variation is the point within a triangle within a circle and square, the sacred delta thus extending its vivifying influence through the whole of created nature:

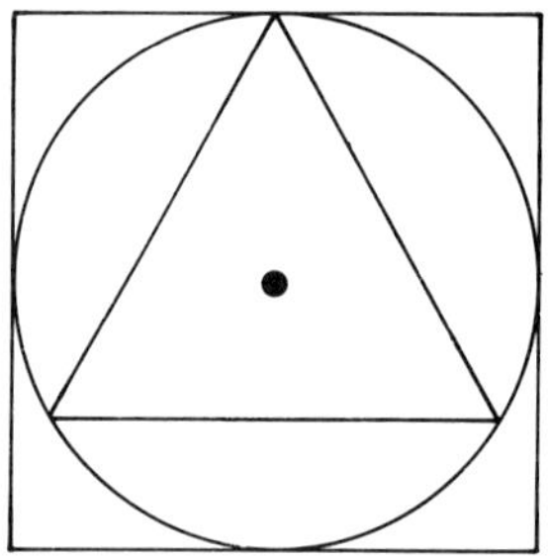

Such metaphysical speculations reached their peak in the Hebrew Qabalah:

This commences with, at its apex, the unknowable, the Ain, the Ain Soph and the Ain Soph Aur, the three veils of negative existence, manifest as the first Sephiroth (or 'Power behind the Throne') Kether. Kether sends out from itself a ray, Fohat, which materializes on a slightly more concrete level as Chokmah to find embodyment in the female matrix as Binah. These Three-in-One represent the spiritual force which can now begin to spread

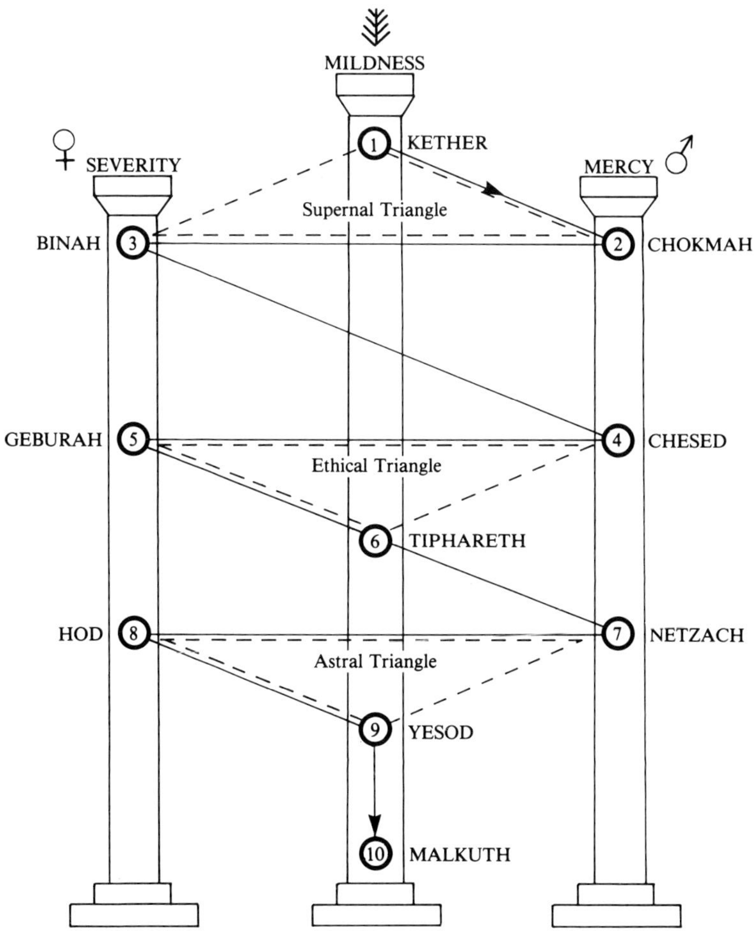
MILDNESS
SEVERITY
MERCY
KETHER
Supernal Triangle
BINAH
CHOKMAH
GEBURAH
CHESED
Ethical Triangle
TIPHARETH
HOD
NETZACH
Astral Triangle
YESOD
MALKUTH
1
2
3
4
5
6
7
8
9
10

downwards into ever-more material form, through the etheric planes of the fourth to seventh Sephiroth into the Astral and then, finally, to the pure material as Malkuth.

This is a very sketchy outline of a very deep subject, but my aim is not to teach the principles of occult philosophy but to show the close relationship between many different schools and approaches.

To carry on just a little way further with the Qabalah, the superior or supernal triangle could be equated with the Yang forces of Heaven being showered down upon the earth ∧ whilst the inferior or astral triangle could be equated with the Yin forces of earth ∨ — or, equally, Man with his arms uplifted in prayer to receive the forces from heaven \V/. Combine the two triangles, and we have ✡, the six-pointed star or 'Seal of Solomon' — that sigil which purportedly gave that great ruler domination over the spirits of the elements — Earth, Air, Fire and Water.

The two side pillars likewise have significance as the two pillars at the porchway or entrance of King Solomon's Temple, and all three stand also for Wisdom, Strength and Beauty. The central pillar, reaching from Malkuth to the apex or Godhead can also represent the Tree and the principle of the crucifixion, death and rebirth, centred as it is on the sixth Sephiroth, Tiphareth, whose titles in Qabalistic nomenclature bear this out — from the point of view of Kether it is a child, from that of Malkuth it is a King, and from the point of view of the transmutation of force it is a sacrificed god.

The Hindu scriptures are remarkably similar. We have already mentioned the triad of Brahma, Vishnu and Siva — this is also illustrated by the material attributes of:

BRAHMA 'I' (Neutral Energy)
Air or Vayu

SIVA	VISHNU
Fire (Yang) Agni	Water (Yin) Jula

from which all is supposed to have sprung.

The Creator is useless without the Preserver or the Destroyer.
Fire cannot burn without Air; Water cannot move without Air. (It becomes stagnant.)
Life is Wood. (Combination of Air and Water.)
Fire destroys, to give birth to Metal.

The order of Cosmic Evolution acording to Samkhya opinion is:

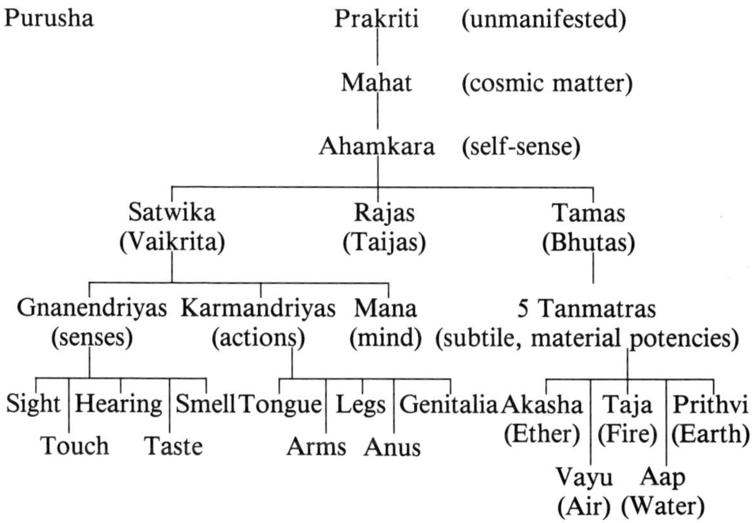

The whole essence of this approach can be summed up in one statement which I find extremely apposite and magnificent in its simplicity: 'God lies sleeping in the Mineral, dreaming in the Vegetable, stirring in the Animal and waking in the Human.'

For an understanding of the basic Chinese approach, I cannot do better than quote Joseph Needham (*Science and Civilisation in China*, Vol. 2):

> Western philosophers laid down as a basic principle of thought that a thing cannot both be and not be at the same time. Chinese philosophers, on the other hand, laid down that a thing is always 'becoming' or 'de-becoming'; all the time on its way to being something else.

For the Chinese, the Tao was all. Tao simply means 'the way', or 'the Path' (the Chinese character is made up of the sign for 'head' and the sign for 'going'), and yet the Tao *was*. It existed in and of itself, with no beginning and no end. It was the true uroborus, the archetypical mandala, carrying within itself the union of the two opposites, and yet it contained in itself its own pathways of self-perception — it existed apart from its percipient, yet the percipient was a part of it, as was the very act of his perception and understanding. It was the Way, yet it was its own beginning and end.

> The Tao gave birth to the One; the One gave birth successively to two things, three things, up to ten thousand. These ten thousand creatures cannot turn their backs to the shade without having the sun on their bellies, and it is upon this blending of the breaths that their harmony depends.
> — *Tao Teh Ching* (Chapter XLII of Arthur Waley's translation)

That beginning was once again the unknowable, the Tai I:

> We say that there was a great Principle of Change (Tai I), a great Origin (Tai ch'u), a great Beginning (Tai shih) and a great Primordial Undifferentiatedness (Tai su). At the great Change, ch'i was not yet manifest. At the great Origin, ch'i began to exist. At the great Beginning came the beginning of form and shape. In the great Primordial Undifferentiatedness lay the beginning of matter. When ch'i, shapes and matter, were still indistinguishably blended together, that state is called chaos (hun-lun). All things were mixed in it, and had not yet been separated from one another . . . The purer and lighter elements (ch'ing ch'ing che), tending upwards, made the heavens; the grosser and heavier elements (cho chung che), tending downwards, made the earth . . .
> — Lieh Tzu — fourth century BC (*vide* Needham)

The Tai gave birth to the One, and the Tai I manifest itself in two ways as in the diagram, the Rule of Two, the Yin/Yang which then split into its two halves, Yin and Yang, which then formed the Active and Potential energies which realized themselves on the levels of Heaven, Earth and Man, the Rule of Three. (It will be noticed that on the passage downwards Yin and Yang reverse their positions — this is an illustration showing that all 'matter'

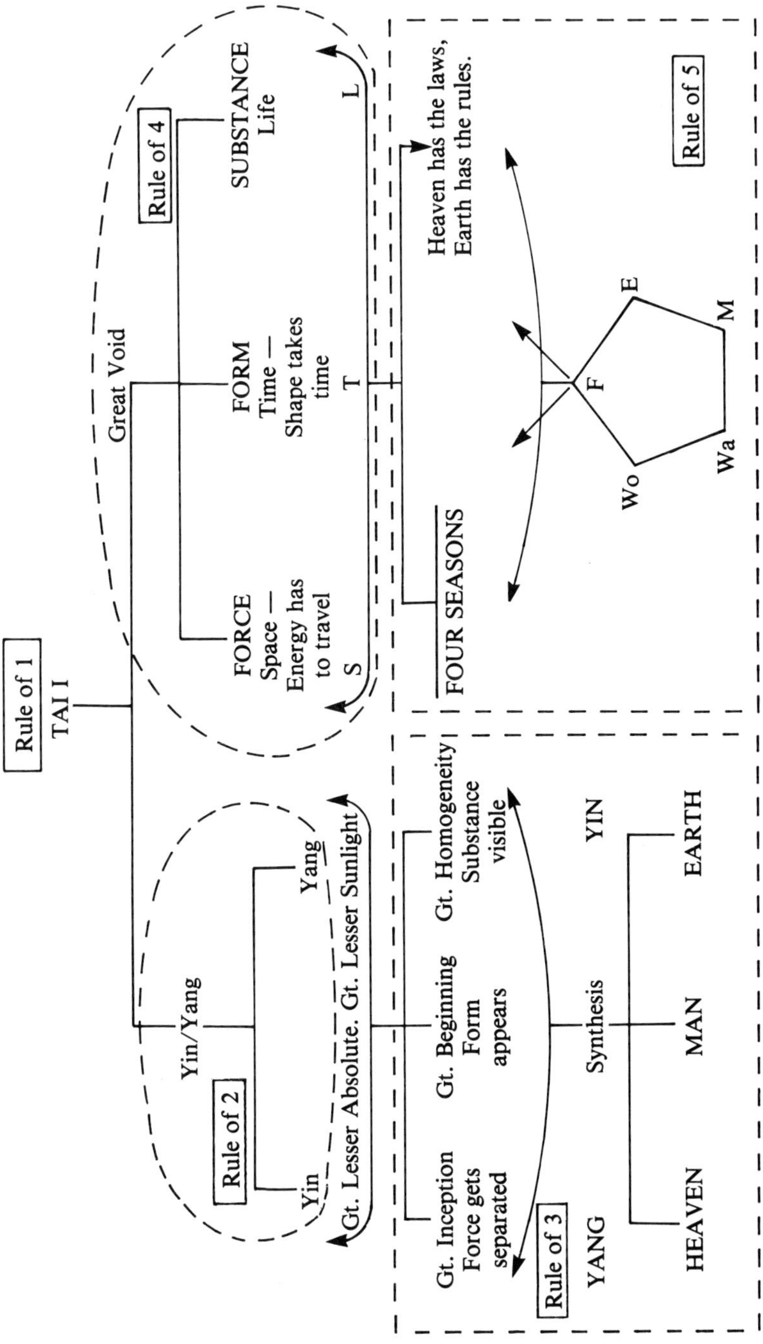
Rule of 1
TAI I
Great Void
Rule of 4
FORCE
Space —
Energy has
to travel
FORM
Time —
Shape takes
time
SUBSTANCE
Life
S
T
L
FOUR SEASONS
Heaven has the laws,
Earth has the rules.
E
M
F
Wo
Wa
Rule of 5
Yin/Yang
Rule of 2
Yin
Yang
Gt. Lesser Absolute. Gt. Lesser Sunlight
Gt. Inception
Force gets
separated
Gt. Beginning
Form
appears
Gt. Homogeneity
Substance
visible
Rule of 3
YANG
Synthesis
YIN
HEAVEN
MAN
EARTH

as presented to the world is an external representation of its inner self which is of opposite polarity — see the concept of the Persona and Anima in psychological theory, or George Osawa's reversal of polarity of the Tsang and Fu organs.) Parallel with these transformations comes the formation of energy itself, manifesting in Space and Time as the Rule of Four — Energy, Space, Time and Life, which gives rise to the four seasons of the year and (the Rule of Five) the Five Elements through which they manifest themselves.

It is stated that an understanding of these five rules can come only in a reverse order, that is, one must be able to feel and comprehend the Rule of Five before one can understand the Rule of Four; one must understand the Rule of Four before one can approach the Rule of Three, the Rule of Three before that of Two, and only then can one begin to comprehend the Tao, or Rule of One. Intuition affirms that when this stage is reached one should no longer need to use the needles . . .

> If one can understand Yin/Yang and Sanjiao one is a Minister,
> If one can reason them out one is a Prince,
> If one can apply them, one is an Emperor,
> But the Sage is respected by the Emperor, because the Sage knows the principle of the Tai I.
>
> The four seasons and Yin and Yang are the beginning and the end of everything, the root of birth and death. If one goes against the rule of this one can get injury, creating general catastrophes, like a flood, which affect all others as well. If one doesn't go against the rule disease doesn't occur, this is the rule of Tao.
>
> — *Su Wen*, Chapter 2

The goal of the Chinese sage was union with the Tai I, as was that of the Hindu mystic in achieving Samadhi. The goal of the Qabalist mystic was the same — to travel from Malkuth to Kether via one of the thirty-two paths of the Qabalah, the most direct route being straight up the central column through the mediator Tiphareth. In like manner, the Hindu Yogi would awaken the sleeping 'Serpent' or Kundalini power of the spinal chahkras, from the sacrum to the top of the head; the lateral columns of the Qabalah have their bodily counterpart in the lateral spinal pathways of Ida and Pingala.

2.
ASTRONOMICAL BACKGROUND

The philosophical sub-stratum was prepared, and in the tableau of the night sky these conceptions took on the appearance of reality . . .

Looking upwards into the heavens the observer perceived one fixed, immovable star — the Pole star, and this, for him, was the centre of the Tao. Watching through the year, the other constellations moved majestically upwards in a clockwise direction from east to west, marking in their progress the climatic changes through the seasons, and the changes in the Yin/Yang balance which is the essence of the Tao.

In his mind he pictured Yang as a dragon — the distillation of Fire and Life, of warmth and activity, and with the coming of Spring the dragon beneath the earth was stirring and warming the soil with its breath, and in the sky he observed the first appearance of the tip of the horn of the young dragon in the rising of the star Arcturus in the east. And as the sun set in the west to close the day, so the moon rose in the east to open the night, and when the full moon appeared in the east exactly opposite the sunset in the west, and to the right of Arcturus, that was the last full moon of the old year.

Slowly the dragon emerged from his winter's sleep, and the second horn, symbolized by the star Virgo (Chio) came into view. And when the next full moon appeared with the two stars Arcturus and Virgo to its right, that was the first full moon of the new year, and marked the exact moment of the beginning of spring.

(Symbolically, 'the dragon carries the full moon in its mouth', and in the famous Dragon Dance, heralding the Chinese New Year, we see the dragon with the ball in front of it which is emblematic of this event.)

The dragon mounts higher. The star Antares, corresponding to his heart, appears, coinciding with the third full moon and also the appearance of the constellation Orion in the west, and the Yang reaches its climax with summer and then slowly decreases. The wheeling constellations mark the passage of the year, and when Orion has passed over into the east and the heart of the dragon (Yang) has begun to decline in the west, Yang has begun to become Yin, and the ninth full moon heralds the beginning of autumn.

By the use of a gnomon — a vertical pole — to measure the length of the sun's shadow by day to determine the solstices, and the transits of the stars by night to observe the revolutions of the sidereal year, there were very precise methods of determining the exact beginnings of the specific seasons (noting that the solstices and equinoxes marked the middle of the seasons and not their beginnings).

The twelve full moons gave the exact divisions of the year, together with the relative state of the Yin and Yang heavenly influences. The four quarters of the year were known as the 'Palaces of the Seasons' — thus there was the 'Palace of Spring', the 'Palace of Summer', the 'Palace of Autumn' and the 'Palace of Winter'. The Pole Star, around which all revolved, was called the 'Central Palace', and represented the Tao itself which engendered the Yin/Yang manifestations.

The determination of the seasons was fixed by a study of those stars which rise in the east and then decline in the west, but there are others which do not disappear below the horizon but rotate around the Pole Star in an opposite direction, from west to east. Amongst these, the most prominent is that constellation known in the Western world as the Plough, which has a 24-hour cycle of rotation. If it were directly above the Pole Star at 00.00-hours it would be due east at 06.00-hours, directly below at 12.00-hours, and due west at 18.00-hours. However, this rotation advances by 4 minutes every day, so that in three months it has advanced by 6 hours, which means that three months later it is due east at 00.00-hours, directly below at 06.00-hours, etc., thus providing a yearly measurement as well as an hourly one.

Chaumfrault writes:

> At the moment Arcturus rises, looking at the sky at 18.00-hours, to the NE the full moon appears, and also the Plough in the NE. Arcturus is in the direct prolongation of the last two stars — the Handle — of the Plough. The Horn of the Dragon, Arcturus, and the direction of the Plough indicate the beginning of spring. Six weeks later the two signs appear not in the NE but directly in the east, and mark the Spring Equinox which is the centre of the Palace of Spring.

The other seasons are marked by the appearance of their own specific constellations, determined by similar principles. The Chinese New Year is based upon the appearance of the second new moon after the winter solstice, and varies between 21 January and 19 February.

There is an excerpt from the *Chou Lei* (Record of the Rites of Chou — Han dynasty) quoted by Needham which enumerates the duties of the Imperial Astronomer (Feng Hsiang Shih):

> He concerns himself with the twelve years (the sidereal revolution of Jupiter), the twelve months, the twelve (double-) hours, the ten days, and the position of the 28 stars (the determinative stars of the Hsiu). He distinguishes them and orders them so that he can make a general plan of the state of the heavens. He takes observations of the sun at the winter and summer solstices, and of the moon at the spring and autumn equinoxes, in order to determine the succession of the four seasons.

It is to be expected that, to such acute observers, the presence and movements of the planets would be considered of interest and import, and the cycle of the planet Jupiter must have attracted early attention because of its twelve year (actually 11.86) periodicity, which would correlate with the twelve months of the year.

The months of the year had specific names, and an animal, supposed to exemplify by its nature the character of the month, assigned to each. These are also the names of the twelve Terrestrial Branches. (See *Table 2* overleaf.)

Rat	Tzu
Ox	Chou
Tiger	Yin
Hare	Mao
Dragon	Chen
Snake	Si
Horse	Wu
Sheep	Wei
Monkey	Shen
Rooster	Yu
Dog	Shu
Pig	Hai

Table 2.

Each of the years of the twelve-yearly Jupiter cycle was given the same name, but each year would also correlate with the positions of certain of 28 stars (hsiu) in the four Palaces.

For the sake of completion, the stars were:

PALACE		Chinese Name	Star
EASTERN	1	Chio	α Virginis
Blue	2	Khang	κ Virginis
Dragon	3	Ti	α^2 Librae
	4	Fang	π Scorpii
	5	Hsin	σ Scorpii
	6	Wei	μ^1 Scorpii
	7	Chi	γ Sagittarii
NORTHERN	8	Nan Too	ϕ Sagittarii
Black	9	Niu	β Capricornii
Tortoise	10	Nü	ϵ Aquarii
	11	Hsü	β Aquarii
	12	Wei	α Aquarii
	13	Shih	α Pegasi
	14	Pi	γ Pegasi

PALACE		Chinese Name		Star
WESTERN	15	Khuei	η	Andromeda
White	16	Lou	β	Arietis
Tiger	17	Wei	$\psi\iota$	Arietis
	18	Mao	η	Tauri
	19	Pi	ϵ	Tauri
	20	Tsui	λ	Orionis
	21	Shen	χ	Orionis
SOUTHERN	22	Ching	μ	Geminorum
Red	23	Kuei	θ	Cancri
Bird	24	Liu	δ	Hydrae
	25	Hsing	α	Hydrae
	26	Chang	μ	Hydrae
	27	I	α	Crateris
	28	Chen	γ	Corvi

Table 3.

The Central Palace consists of the circumpolar stars ('The Emperor and his Officials').

The system of Hsiu dates back to the fourteenth century BC, and can be found on oracle-bones of the reign of the Emperor Wu-Ting.

The corresponding months were:

	Month	Associated Hsiu		Direction
1.	Tzu	Nü, Hsu, Wei	(10,11,12)	North
2.	Chou	Tou, Niu	(8,9)	North
3.	Yin	Wei, Chi	(6,7)	East
4.	Mao	Ti, Fang, Hsin	(3,4,5)	East
5.	Chen	Chio, Khang	(1,2)	East
6.	Si	I, Chen	(27,28)	South
7.	Wu	Liu, Hsing, Chang	(24,25,26)	South
8.	Wei	Ching, Kuei	(22,23)	South
9.	Shen	Tsui, Shen	(20,21)	West
10.	Yu	Wei, Mao, Pi	(17,18,19)	West
11.	Shu	Khuei, Lou	(15,16)	West
12.	Hai	Shih, Pi	(13,14)	North

Table 4.

I have just mentioned the giving of the names of animals to the specific months. The corresponding years, as we have seen, were given the same names and had the same animals allocated to them — a feature well-known to any who have looked at a book on Chinese astrology. The seasons were also symbolized by zoological attributes as follows:

> Spring was a Green Dragon — the rising Yang in the East.
> Summer was a Red Bird — a quail or, later, a Phoenix, rising every year in golden glory from the ashes of its own self-immolation.
> Autumn was a White Tiger, which descended fierce from the hills in autumn.
> Winter was a Black Turtle, which was cold-blooded and liked the damp.

Through the ages various extensions and changes in the symbolism took place, until eventually the present day schema was arrived at:

S
(Summer)

Horse

Snake Sheep

Dragon Monkey

E (Spring) Hare Rooster W (Autumn)

Tiger Dog

Ox Pig

Rat

N
(Winter)

(When Buddhism came to China and attempted to supplant Taoism a legend became extant that when the Buddha lay dying he summoned all the animals to him, the first twelve to arrive being, in order of appearance, the Rat, Ox, Tiger, Hare, Dragon, Snake, Horse, Sheep, Monkey, Rooster, Dog and Pig, and that as a reward they were immortalized in the seasons. This bears no relationship to the symbolic qualities of the animals which explains why they were chosen to fill their respective positions.)

We have considered briefly how the monthly, seasonal, yearly and twelve-yearly cycles were conceived. There is yet one further cycle to mention, and that is the sixty-year one.

Once in every sixty years the moon, earth, sun and Pole Star lie in the same line, and the Chinese calendar starts at the occulting:

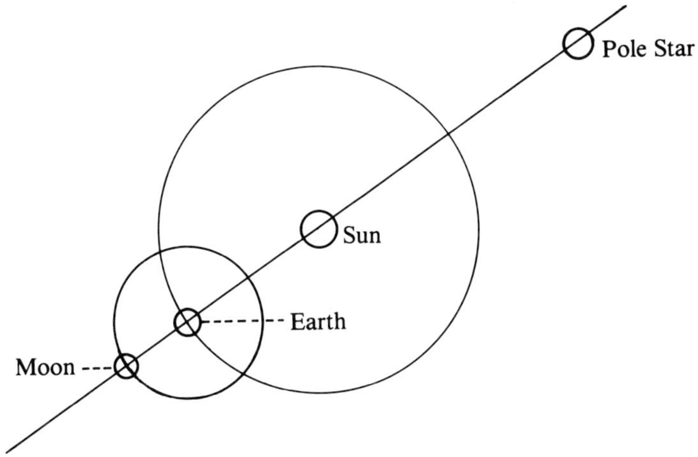

3.

THE 'GREAT' OR SIXTY-YEAR CYCLE

'T'ien Tao Yu Tu'
(The Tao of Heaven has its regular, measured movements)

The revolving heavens gave an idea of the relative Yang or Yin influences being poured down upon the earth from the celestial source — spring was the beginning of Yang, summer was Yang maximum; with the decline of summer came the decline of Yang and the increment of Yin, which in its turn reached its maximum in the winter to slowly decline and in its turn give way to the advent of Yang in the spring once more.

It will be seen that this is in correlation with the 5-Phases or so-called 5-Elements:

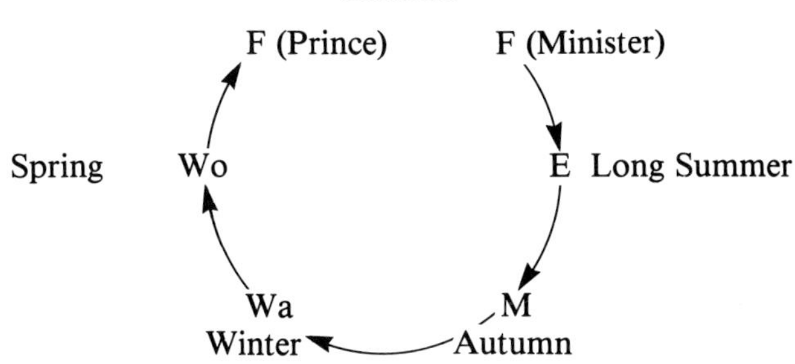

Each of the 5-Phases has a climatic influence associated with it, and it is natural that these should be regarded as the atmospheric (or celestial) energies which could affect the earth:

Heat
F

Wind Wo E Humidity

Wa M
Cold Dryness

But the essence of Chinese philosophy is reciprocity — a constant interplay between opposites. The celestial energies were regarded as basically Yang in nature, to be balanced by the basically Yin energies of earth, which constantly reacted with them. The Yin energies of earth were governed by the daily, monthly and yearly cycles of the sun and were the twelve Terrestrial Branches represented in Man by the constantly evolving Ch'i energy in the meridians, the 6 Chiaos. These were thought to manifest in an evolving Yin and Yang pattern, in the order Shao Yin (Little Yin), Tai Yin (Great Yin), Shao Yang (Little Yang), Yang Ming (Bright Yang), Tai Yang (Great Yang), Jueh Yin (Decreasing Yin), Shao Yin (Little Yin), Tai Yin (Great Yin) . . . in a constantly revolving cycle.

Each one of the twelve divisions of the year was assigned to one of the branches, starting with the Little Yin in the North:

Month	**Name**	**Branch**	
Rat	Tzu	Shao Yin	Yin
Ox	Chou	Tai Yin	
Tiger	Yin	Shao Yang	
Hare	Mao	Yang Ming	Yang
Dragon	Chen	Tai Yang	
Snake	Si	Jueh Yin	
Horse	Wu	Shao Yin	Yin
Sheep	Wei	Tai Yin	
Monkey	Shen	Shao Yang	
Rooster	Yu	Yang Ming	Yang
Dog	Shu	Tai Yang	
Pig	Hai	Jueh Yin	Yin

Table 5.

And just as the branches show a cyclical evolution from Yin to Yang and back again, so the celestial influences also manifest in an alternating Yang-Yin pattern. These celestial influences — the Ten Celestial Stems — are the same as the 5-Elements, but instead of the creative cycle starting with Wood the cycle runs Earth, Metal, Water, Wood, Fire. We have said that they observe an alternating Yang-Yin pattern, and this is as follows:

Chia	Earth	(Strong-Yang)
Yee	Metal	(Weak-Yin)
Ping	Water	(Strong-Yang)
Ding	Wood	(Weak-Yin)
Wu	Fire	(Strong-Yang)
Ji	Earth	(Weak-Yin)
Geng	Metal	(Strong-Yang)
Shin	Water	(Weak-Yin)
Ren	Wood	(Strong-Yang)
Gui	Fire	(Weak-Yin)

Table 6.

It will be seen that the 5-Phase cycle has to occur twice in order to make up the required number of ten, and that the character of the element alters the second time round so that although Chia Earth is strong and Yang, Ji Earth is weak and Yin.

* * *

Man is the result of the constant interplay between the forces of Heaven and Earth, and those forces are acting the whole of the time. Just as there are inherent biological rhythms within him responding to daily and yearly rhythms, so the interplay between the Celestial Stems and the Terrestrial Branches occurs on constantly changing temporal levels and permutations. There is the daily effect upon his meridial energies and the 24-hour cycle; there is a seasonal effect via the cycle of the months, and there is a deeper effect via the 12-yearly cycle (which could possibly equate very roughly with that of the sun-spots). The terrestrial level is all on a cycle of twelve, the celestial level is all on a cycle of ten.

By successively pairing each with each, we arrive at the following table.

	Stem	Branch		Stem	Branch		Stem	Branch
1.	Chia	Tzu	21.	Chia	Shen	41.	Chia	Chen
2.	Yee	Chou	22.	Yee	Yu	42.	Yee	Si
3.	Ping	Yin	23.	Ping	Shu	43.	Ping	Wu
4.	Ding	Mao	24.	Ding	Hai	44.	Ding	Wei
5.	Wu	Chen	25.	Wu	Tzu	45.	Wu	Shen
6.	Ji	Si	26.	Ji	Chou	46.	Ji	Yu
7.	Geng	Wu	27.	Geng	Yin	47.	Geng	Shu
8.	Shin	Wei	28.	Shin	Mao	48.	Shin	Hai
9.	Ren	Shen	29.	Ren	Chen	49.	Ren	Tzu
10.	Gui	Yu	30.	Gui	Si	50.	Gui	Chou
11.	Chia	Shu	31.	Chia	Wu	51.	Chia	Yin
12.	Yee	Hai	32.	Yee	Wei	52.	Yee	Mao
13.	Ping	Tzu	33.	Ping	Shen	53.	Ping	Chen
14.	Ding	Chou	34.	Ding	Yu	54.	Ding	Si
15.	Wu	Yin	35.	Wu	Shu	55.	Wu	Wu
16.	Ji	Mao	36.	Ji	Hai	56.	Ji	Wei
17.	Geng	Chen	37.	Geng	Tzu	57.	Geng	Shen
18.	Shin	Si	38.	Shin	Chou	58.	Shin	Yu
19.	Ren	Wu	39.	Ren	Yin	59.	Ren	Shu
20.	Gui	Wei	40.	Gui	Mao	60.	Gui	Hai

Table 7.

It will be seen that it takes a total of sixty possible combinations before the cycle repeats itself with Chia-Tzu. This conforms to the great-cycle of sixty years if we are dealing with yearly influences, and also to the 5-Element influence on the twelve branches ($5 \times 12 = 60$) if we are considering the daily cycles.

The Stems are the celestial energies given out, and the Branches are the reacting energies of earth, each year being characterized by the combination of the two.

The current 60-year cycle commenced in the year 1924, which would therefore be number 1, or a year governed by the Stem Chia and the Branch Tzu, therefore known as a Chia-Tzu year. 1925 would be a Yee-Chou year, and 1980 would be the 57th in the cycle — a Geng-Shen year. The next cycle commences with a Chia-Tzu year in 1984.

The whole may be conveniently shown in tabular form as:

STEMS

BRANCHES				Chia E +	Yee M −	Ping Wa +	Ding Wo −	Wu F +	Ji E −	Geng M +	Shin Wa −	Ren Wo +	Gui F −
Rat	Tzu	Shao Yin	F + (Prince)	1924 1984		1936 1996		1948 2008		1960 2020		1972 2032	
Ox	Chou	Tai Yin	E −		1925 1985		1937 1997						
Tiger	Yin	Shao Yang	F + (Minister)	1974		1926 1986		1938 1998					
Hare	Mao	Yang Ming	M −				1927 1987		1939 1999				
Dragon	Chen	Tai Yang	Wa +	1964				1928 1988		1940 2000			
Snake	Si	Jueh Yin	Wo −						1929 1989		1941 2001		
Horse	Wu	Shau Yin	F + (Prince)	1954				1978		1930 1990		1942 2002	
Sheep	Wei	Tai Yin	E −								1931 1991		1943 2003
Monkey	Shen	Shao Yang	F + (Minister)	1944 2004				1968				1932 1992	
Rooster	Yu	Yang Ming	M −		1945 2005								1933 1993
Dog	Shu	Tai Yang	Wa +	1934 1994		1946 2006		1958					
Pig	Hai	Jueh Yin	Wo −		1935 1995		1947 2007						1983 2043

Table 8.

The Stems are used to calculate the movements, and the Branches the energies, that is, the Yang of Heaven is the basic motivating force whilst the Yin Branches of Earth are the resultant energies springing from that motivation. The basic force behind a specific year is therefore that determined by the Celestial Stem of that year, i.e., 1940 was Metal, 1942 was Wood, but how that force will manifest itself is determined by the Terrestrial Branch.

The more immediate characteristics of the year are those of the atmospheric influences attributed to the concerned elements and Chiaos. (See *Table 9* overleaf.)

Stems:	E	= Humid	— Receives the seed and gives the crop.
	M	= Dryness	— Obeys the hand of the worker and takes different forms.
	Wa	= Dampness	— Wets and descends.
	Wo	= Wind	— Is pliable; bends and straightens.
	F	= Heat	— Burns and ascends.

Branches:	Shao Yin	= Fire Prince +	= Fire
	Tai Yin	= E −	= Dampness
	Shao Yang	= Fire Minister +	= Heat
	Yang Ming	= M −	= Dryness
	Tai Yang	= Wa +	= Cold
	Jueh Yin	= Wo −	= Wind

Table 9. 'Great Rule' of Chou King.

If one looks at Table 9 one will see that on both Stems and Branches, Yin and Yang, weakness and strength, alternate. Thus on the Stems we can have an E+ (Chia), or an E− (Ji), but on the Branches the terrestrial influences are constant, with M always weak and Wa always strong.

The resultant condition is always dependent upon the balance between Heaven and Earth. Although the Stems are the celestial motivating movements, they are also the recipients of the earthly energies; although the Branches are the resultant energies of earth, they are also the recipients of the celestial energies. (That is why one or two writers have confused the issue by referring to the Stems as terrestrial energies and to the Branches as celestial!) But Heaven is Yang and Earth is Yin, and harmony on earth is the result of the balance between the two forces. If the energy of Heaven should predominate there will be Yang-type problems; if that of the Earth should be in excess then the problems will be of a Yin-type.

Referring back to Table 9, we can thus determine the basic character of any particular year. A Stem sign of M+ will mean an underlying tendency for dryness, modified by the Branch, i.e., M+ with Shao Yang (Heat) means a hot, dry year; with the Tai Yang (cold) a cold, dry year. But the Shao Yang, apart from its atmospheric influence of heat, is also Fire+, and Fire and Metal are opposed on the Ko cycle. In this case both influences are + and so, although it will be a hot, dry year, the F+ will tend to dominate. The F+ is the Branch aspect and the Branches are Yin, therefore the excessive heat will cause Yin-type problems. In this instance we are talking about a Geng-Yin (or Geng-Shen) year. If it were a Yee-Yin or a Yee-Shen year, with M−, then the destructive effect of the F+ would be even stronger. In the second instance where the Branch aspect was the Tai Yang, this is Water +. The Stem is Metal and the Branch is Water; the Stem is mother to the Branch on the Sheng cycle and the influence is favourable — the year will therefore be basically dry but colder than usual, and as the energies are harmonious there will be no overt atmospheric disturbances.

Favourable influences are either identicals or Mother/Son; unfavourable are Reverse Sheng (where the Son is strong and the Mother weak), Ko, or Wu (reverse Ko) cycle.

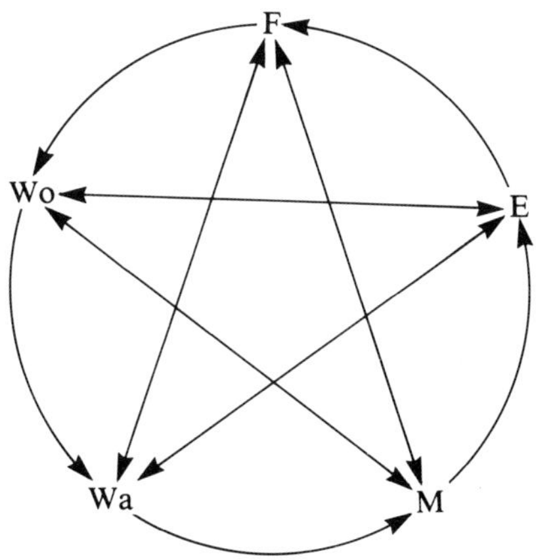

As we are dealing here with the 'Great Cycle' or yearly influences, there will not be such a marked effect on the physiological energy as would pertain on the seasonal or daily cycles, but the underlying correspondencies are always present and a year which placed, say E−, in an unfavourable aspect (possibly opposed by Wo+) could be a year in which tendencies to spleen or stomach problems would manifest themselves.

Earlier on we noted that the influence of the Stems could be characterized as either + or −, an excess or deficiency of energy. In the case of an excess, this will be sufficient to overcome, or ameliorate, the adverse effect of an opposing energy, and will also affect the years on either side of it. Because of the alternation of Yin and Yang in the yearly cycle, a Yang (strong) year must necessarily have a Yin (weak) year both preceding and succeeding it, and it will therefore tend to overcome their influence. This means that its own influence will both arrive early and last longer — possibly by about thirteen days at each end. For harmony to be achieved the energies should really arrive exactly at their appointed time. If they arrive late it is because they are too weak, if early, because they are too strong. This will cause various imbalances and, in nature, calamities such as earthquakes or floods and storms, depending upon the element involved (i.e., Earth, storms and floods; Metal, dryness of vegetation; Water, clouded skies and cold; Wood, wind and tempest; Fire, extreme heat). In man there would be a tendency for diseases in the associated organs.

Where there is a deficiency its specific quality would tend to be affected by those of the preceding and succeeding years, whilst it would also suffer from a weakness on the Ko cycle effect — for example, a weakness of Fire would render it liable to be attacked by the cold of Water, and the year would be cold with little growth.

> When the year of Wood is in excess, the energy of wind will flow and the spleen of Earth will suffer. People will suffer from diarrhoea with undigested foods, decreased appetite, weight loss, depression, abdominal rumbling, abdominal swelling and swelling of limbs. And Jupiter in the sky will be bright (due to excess of Wood year).
>
> In severe cases, people may become dizzy and jumpy, blurred vision and the disease of the head (due to upsurging energy of the liver). The energy of earth fails to perform its administrative duty (due to inhibition exercised by the energy of wind), the energy of life (namely, the energy of wind) becomes a lone ruler, clouds and things flow all over, grasses and trees remain insecure or begin to shake and fall, and people suffer from pain in ribs and vomiting, and when the connective meridian is exhausted, the person will die. And Venus in the sky will be bright (due to excess of liver).
>
> When the year of Fire is in excess, flames and summer heat will be widespread, and the lungs of metal will suffer. People will be under the attack of malaria, scanty energy, cough and asthma, vomiting of blood, discharge of blood from anus, diarrhoea, dry throat, deafness, hot sensations in the middle region, hot sensations around the shoulders and back. And Mars will be bright (due to excess of fire).
>
> In severe cases, people will be under the attack of chest pain,

swelling in the ribs region, pain in the ribs, pain on the sides of chest, back, scapula regions, pain inside the two arms, hot sensations in the body with pain in bones and moist itch. The harvest energy fails to perform its functions and the long energy alone is in the region, so that rains, water, frost, cold will become dominant (in order to control fire). And Mercury will be bright (due to excess of water) in the sky.

If the little Yin and the little Yang are present in the upper region (because hot energy rules on top of the little Yin and fire energy rules on top of the little Yang), fire will be widespread, water will be exhausted and dried up, things will become withered, and people will suffer from hot symptoms such as talking in dreams and insanity, cough and asthma with noisy respiration, diarrhoea with blood; and when the lung meridian is exhausted, the patient will die. And Mars will be bright in the sky . . .

— *Su Wen*, Chapter 69. (Dr Henry Lu's translation)

4.
THE YEARLY CYCLE

The fore-going effects of the 60-year cycle (the Tai Yün or Great Cycle) are, however, far too vague for practical usage. They determine basic underlying characteristics for the whole year, but these are modified to a considerable extent by the more mutable effects of the seasons — the Chu Yün.

The names of the Stems remain the same, but they now govern the energies of the five seasons of the year in the familiar 5-Element picture starting with the Wood of Spring, yet they still follow an alternating Yang-Yin pattern:

Spring	Wood	Yang	Chia
		Yin	Yee
Summer	Fire	Yang	Ping
		Yin	Ding
Long Summer	Earth	Yang	Wu
		Yin	Ji
Autumn	Metal	Yang	Geng
		Yin	Shen
Winter	Water	Yang	Ren
		Yin	Gui

Table 10.

These are known as 'Host' energies and are unchangeable, being the basic seasonal influences, but they are superimposed upon the fundamental substrata of the yearly energies, and the resultant effects are known as 'Guest' energies.

The spring of the year is governed by the unchanging Great Cycle aspect of the year, and if we place this in the centre we can then draw around it the seasonal influences, starting with Wood for spring:

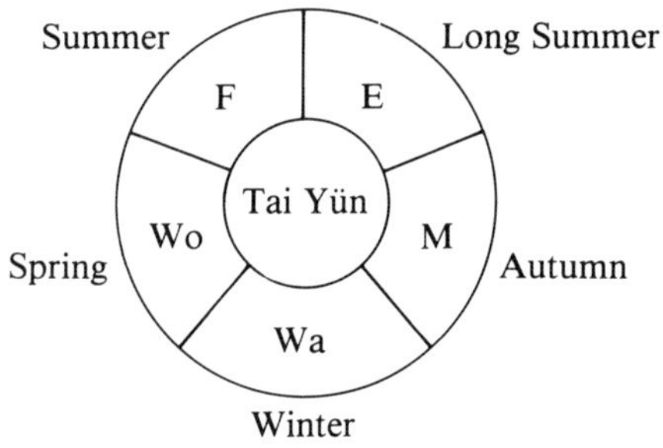

We can then add a further ring showing the spring element corresponding to the stem of the specific year (as shown in Table 8 in the previous chapter), taking the first five stems as an example:

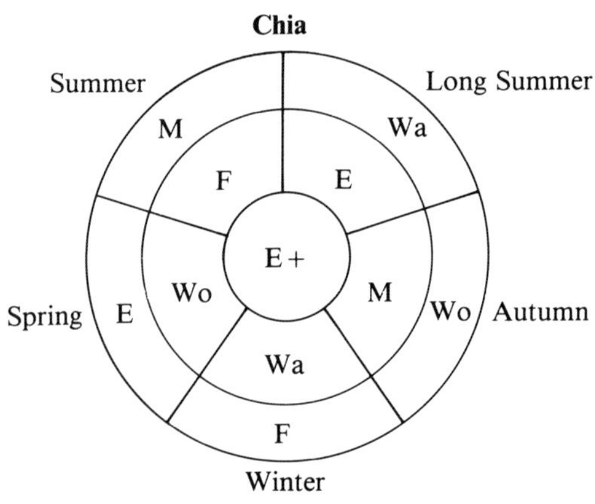

Yee

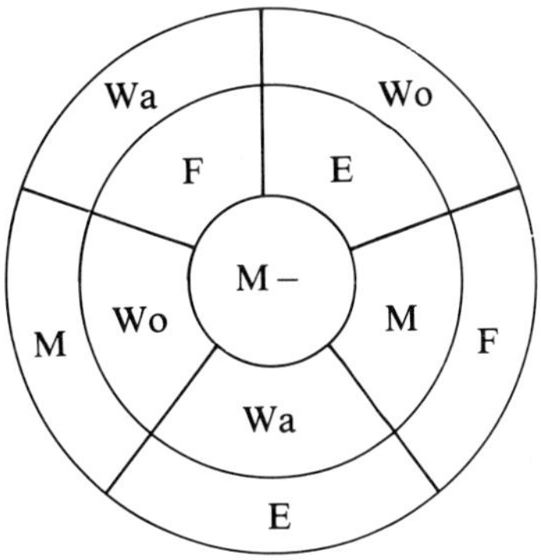

Ping

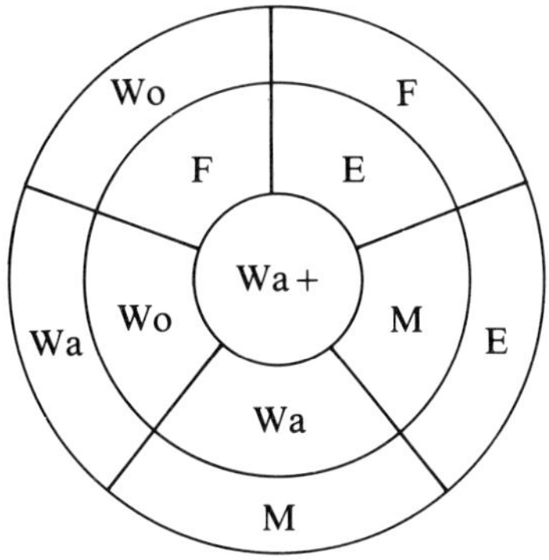

Ding

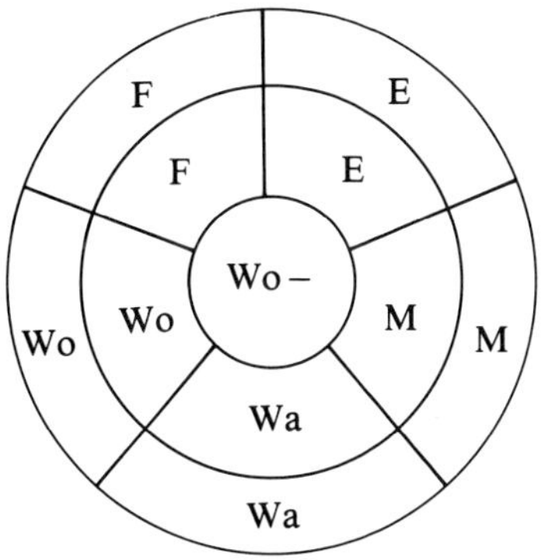

Wu

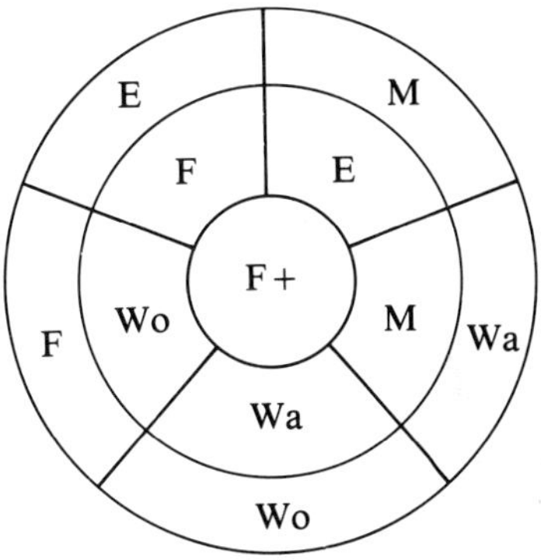

What we have done is place the corresponding stem of the Tai Yün in the centre — e.g., Chia (see Table 8) is E +, Yee is M –, etc. The second circle remains constant — these are the normal elemental influences for the seasons. The third or outer circle takes its spring element from the Tai Yün, e.g., in a Chia year the spring element is E, in a Yee year it is Metal. We will notice that the outer circle rotates one division anti-clockwise at each New Year or change of Tai Yün, and also that apart from every fourth, or Wood year, the influences are quite mixed. Taking the first year, or Chia, as an example, the underlying influence is Earth, or humidity, but spring, which is usually Wind, is also characterized by Earth humidity, so the spring will be more humid than usual, with possible spleen and stomach troubles. The autumn (dry) with an Earth (humid) substratum and a Wood (windy) dominating guest energy will be slightly more humid and windy than usual. In the second or Yee year the autumn, usually dry, would be considerably hotter and drier than usual, because of the underlying influence of Metal — further dryness — and the dominance of the guest energy of Fire.

As with the Great Cycle, the Celestial Stems of the annual cycle are in their turn balanced by the Terrestrial Branches, and these reflect the effect of the celestial movements on the seasonal energies. They are linked to the heavenly cycles by the division of the year into twenty-four 'fortnightly' periods (actually of 15.21 days each):

	Designation	**Beginning:**	**Step**	
1.	Great Cold	January 21	1	Rising
2.	Beginning of Spring	February 5		
3.	The Rains	February 20		
4.	Awakening from Hibernation	March 7		
5.	Spring Equinox	March 22	2	
6.	Clear and Bright (Weather)	April 6		
7.	Rain on the Grains	April 21		
8.	Beginning of Summer	May 6		
9.	Lesser Fullness (of Grain)	May 22	3	
10.	Grain in Ear	June 7		
11.	Summer Solstice	June 22		
12.	Lesser Heat	July 8		
13.	Great Heat	July 24	4	Declining
14.	Beginning of Autumn	August 8		
15.	End of Heat	August 24		
16.	White Dew	September 8		
17.	Autumn Equinox	September 24	5	
18.	Cold Dew	October 9		
19.	Descent of Hoar Frost	October 24		
20.	Beginning of Winter	November 8		
21.	Lesser Snow	November 23	6	
22.	Great Snow	December 7		
23.	Winter Solstice	December 22		
24.	Lesser Cold	January 6		

Table 11.

If these twenty-four periods are sub-divided into groups of six we arrive once more at correlation with the 6 Chiaos, but in a different order to correspond to the seasonal influences pertaining:

Division	**Chiao**	
1	Jueh Yin	Wood (Wind)
2	Shao Yin	Fire Prince (Fire)
3	Shao Yang	Fire Minister (Heat)
4	Tai Yin	Earth (Humidity)
5	Yang Ming	Metal (Dryness)
6	Tai Yang	Water (Cold)

Table 12.

These are the Host energies of the Terrestrial Branches, and they in their turn have Guest energies which are the result of the effect of the Stem movements on the Host energies. This entails the Chiao governing the year as a whole, which is known as the 'Heavenly Governed Chiao' (Szu-t'ien chih ch'i) being selected as the main Guest Chiao — to find which this is, again refer to Table 8 given in the previous chapter, where the Chiaos pertaining to the specific Branches are tabulated. As an example, 1979 was a Ji-Wei year, and the Chiao of the Branch Wei is the Tai Yin, therefore the Tai Yin is the Heavenly Governed Chiao for that year and is the one which exerts the major influence over the whole year, but more especially the first half, when the energy is rising.

This Chiao is assigned to the third of the six divisions, and the remaining divisions of the year have the specific Chiaos associated with the succeeding branches, that is, the third division was Wei, therefore the succeeding divisions would be:

3	Wei	Tai Yin
4	Shen	Shao Yang
5	Yu	Yang Ming
6	Shu	Tai Yang
1	Hai	Jueh Yin
2	Tzu	Shao Yin

As the Heavenly Governed Chiao governs the first half of the year, so the second, declining, half of the year also comes under specific rulership, that of the Chiao of the sixth step. This is called the

'Source Chiao' (Tsai-ch'uan chih ch'i), and in the above example would be the Tai Yang.

It will be seen that whatever Chiaos happen to govern divisions three and six, there will always be a Yin/Yang balance:

Division 3	= Tzu	=	Shao Yin,	6	=	Mao	=	Yang Ming
3	= Chou	=	Tai Yin,	6	=	Chen	=	Tai Yang
3	= Yin	=	Shao Yang,	6	=	Si	=	Jueh Yin
3	= Mao	=	Yang Ming,	6	=	Wu	=	Shao Yin, etc.

The other four Chiaos are called 'Intermediate' (Chien ch'i). The Heavenly Governed Chiao and the Source Chiao are assigned two of these each, thus in the example previously given of a Ji-Wei year:

	Position 3 Tai Yin	
Position 2 Shao Yin		Position 4 Shao Yang
Position 1 Jueh Yin		Position 5 Yang Ming
	Position 6 Tai Yang	

but their influences are subordinate to those of the two major branches. In Chapter 68 of *Su Wen*; the Yellow Emperor asked:

> Could I hear about the abundance and decline of three Yins and three Yangs in relation to the six energies?

Chi Po replied:

> The upper and the lower positions are predetermined, and the left and right sides are regulated according to fixed principles. Therefore, on the right side of the Little Yang, the Bright Yang is in the reign; on the right side of the Bright Yang, the Great Yang is in the reign; on the right side of the Great Yang, the Decreasing Yin is in the reign; on the right side of the Decreasing Yin, the Little Yin is in the reign; on the right side of the Little Yin, the Great Yin is in the reign; on the right side of the Great Yin, the Little Yang is in the reign; such

are the secondary phenomena of energies, and the sage will wait for the arrival of energies by facing South.

The quality of the year will depend upon the relative balance between the Stems and Branches and the interplay between the Guest and Host energies. The good Host should always be subordinate to the wishes of his Guest, but provides the basic background in which his guest can circulate.

Just as we saw in Chapter 3, that the quality of the year could be strengthened or weakened by the interplay of the forces involved, so the quality of the seasons or the months can also be altered — all according to the basic rules of the 5-Phases. Always remembering that, for harmony in the household, the welfare of the Guest should predominate; harmony between Guest and Host is essential. If the Host should be Wood and the Guest energy Earth, then according to the law of the Ko cycle the Host will destroy his Guest and calamity will ensue. If the Guest checks the Host — the so-called 'Torment of Heaven' — it is not quite so bad, but would still result in friction and a tendency to meteorological and other disturbances.

Favourable signs are where either Guest or Host (Stem or Branch) are in a Mother-Son relationship, where one feeds the other on the Sheng cycle. If they should be both of the same sign it is not particularly unfavourable, but the pertaining conditions are likely to be exaggerated and possibly extreme.

So far we have mentioned mainly climatic and meteorological conditions, because it is these which manifest from yearly or seasonal influences — hot or cold, wet or dry, windy or humid — but we must not forget that man reacts internally to the external stimuli, and he reacts by the energies inherent in his meridial system.

The six Chiaos were apportioned their respective branches by virtue of their correspondencies to the six seasonal divisions, but they relate also to their respective meridians and Zang/Fu energies; if the Tai Yin (E –) were the Guest Chiao and it happened to be opposed by a Host Wood, then one could anticipate that any individuals with a tendency to trouble with the lungs or spleen would manifest an exacerbation of that trouble (in this case, as the opposition would be from Wood, it is most likely that it would be the spleen which would suffer, as it is the organ directly affected on the Ko cycle). Similarly, if a Guest Yang Ming (M –) happened to coincide with a Host Earth, his bowels would most likely be reasonably 'happy' and his gastric juices functioning well. If the host Earth was the stem Wu there would be a Yang type influence; if the stem Ji, then there would be a more Yin aspected effect.

5.

THE DAILY CYCLE

'Huang tang, pu huan yao' —
('Change the soup's essence while retaining the water')

* * *

'The energy of Heaven moves downwards and the energy of Earth moves upwards, so that communication of energies takes place in the middle where Man resides.'
— *Su Wen*, Chapter 68

We now come to that part of the whole complex system which has the most direct bearing upon our more day-to-day work as practitioners. The actions, or rather the influences, of the year and the season are not to be denigrated — they are the underlying substratum upon which the more immediate reactions are superimposed — but the activity of the points themselves depends upon the circadian rhythms and the body's daily responses, the actual hourly changes which take place in the ebb and flow of the meridial energy.

The approach is known in Chinese as the Tzu Wu Liu Chu (in Pinyin, Zi Wu Liu Zhu) method, or more fully, the Tzu Wu Liu Chu Liao Fa. Tzu is the time of the hours from 11pm to 1am, Wu the hours from 11am to 1pm, Liu means 'flowing', Chu means 'entering', Liao stand for 'treatment', and Fa for 'technique'. The whole therefore means a technique of treatment by entering the energy when it is flowing at its peak periods.

We have encountered a type of this approach in our early elementary studies of the 24-hour clock and the use of Horary Points. However, to the chagrin of the practitioner we now find that the actual 'opening hours' of the meridians do *not* correspond directly with this — they are based on a more subtle reasoning and foundation, and until this fact is grasped any attempt to understand the *modus operandi* will be futile.

The first rule to remember is that, according to tradition, Yang moves forwards and Yin moves backwards. Therefore the Stems, being Yang by nature, always move forward while, conversely, the Branches, being inherently Yin regardless of whether the Tsang or the Fu are involved, always move backwards.

As stated earlier, the names of the Stems and Branches remain the same but the Stems now pertain to the energies governing the meridians (again in 5-Phase order) and the Branches to the hours of the day:

Days

1	2	3	4	5	6	7	8	9	10
Chia	Yee	Ping	Ding	Wu	Ji	Geng	Shen	Ren	Gui
Wo		F		E		M		Wa	
Yang	Yin	Yang	Yin	Yang	Yin	Yang	Yin	Yang	Yin
GB	Li	SI	Ht	St	Sp	Co	Lu	Bl	Ki

Hours

Tzu	+	23.00-01.00 hours
Chou	–	01.00-03.00 hours
Yin	+	03.00-05.00 hours
Mao	–	05.00-07.00 hours
Chen	+	07.00-09.00 hours
Si	–	09.00-11.00 hours
Wu	+	11.00-13.00 hours
Wei	–	13.00-15.00 hours
Shen	+	15.00-17.00 hours
Yu	–	17.00-19.00 hours
Shu	+	19.00-21.00 hours
Hai	–	21.00-23.00 hours

(+ = Yang; – = Yin)

Table 13.

The two facts of energy flow which have to be borne in mind are:

1. The flow of energy in the 5-Phase cycle as portrayed by the Stems, starting in Wood, which feeds Fire, then Earth, Metal and Water.

2. The flow in the individual meridians, the familiar Tsing, Yong, Yu, Ching, Ho sequence. (I prefer the Wade-Giles for this, as it differentiates the points better.) For the convenience of readers who are more familiar with the Pinyin, the correspondencies are:

	Wade-Giles	**Pinyin**	**English ('Essentials')**	**Shanghai Book**	**Dr Henry Lu**
1.	Tsing	Jing	Well	Well	Welling
2.	Yong	Rong	Spring	Gushing	Outpouring
3.	Yu	Shu	Stream	Transporting	Lake
4.	Ching	Jing	River	Penetrating	Flowing
5.	Ho	He	Sea	Uniting	Terminal

The flow of energy in both Stems and Branches follows the Sheng cycle, but with an alternating Yang-Yin pattern:

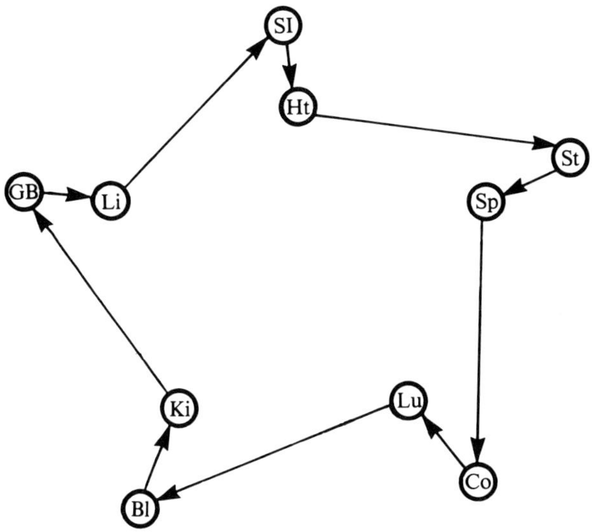

Yang meridians will open only on a Yang day, and Yang points only at a Yang period of time; conversely, Yin meridians will open only on a Yin day, and the points at a Yin period of time. The first day, or 'Head of the Yang Stems', is Chia, and a look at Table 13 will show that this is a GB day. Therefore the GB meridian will open only on a Chia day. We stated that the Branches 'move backwards' — we therefore start at the *end* of the Yang branches, and this is the eleventh period, or Shu. Therefore the GB meridian will begin to open at that time, and the point to open will be its Tsing point, or GB44. We can thus say that GB44 will open on a Chia day at the Shu (19.00-21.00 hours) time.

The next opening *Yang* Stem is Ping, which is SI.

The first point to open on GB days is GB44, which is the Metal point. Metal generates Water, therefore the next point to open would be a Water point, and as this would be on the SI meridian (the next meridian to open), the second point to open would be the Water point (Yong point) of the SI meridian, i.e., SI2.

Although the opening times of the meridians move backwards, the opening of successive points on the cycle moves forwards in time, and SI2 would open at the next Yang period to Chia-Shu, and this would be Yi-Tzu. Thus SI2 opens at the Yi-Tzu time.

I think now is the time to give the table which gives all the opening times with which we are presently concerned, and if the reader follows this with the text he will be able to see how these events, which may seem complicated at first, are actually quite easily worked out. (See *Table 14.*)

The next Yang Stem to open is Wu = St. The previous Yang point was Water — Water generates Wood, so the next point to open would be the Wood point of St, which is St43. The next Yang period is Yin, on the Yee day, so St43 opens at the Yee-Yin time. Successively, the next Yang Stem is Geng (Co); Wood (St43) generates Fire, and the Fire point of Co is Co5, which would open at the next Yang period — Yee-Chen, to be followed by the Earth point of Bladder, Bl54, at Yee-Wu.

We started with the first Stem — Chia. The second Stem, Yee, is Liver. Therefore the next point to open would be the Tsing point of Li, which would open on the Yee day. Remembering that the Branches move backwards, this would open at the first Yin time (Liver is Yin) preceding the Shu time of Gall Bladder, and this is Yu. Thus the point Li1 opens at Yee-Yu.

As in our previous example, the next point opens on a Ding day and is Heart (next Yin Stem after Liver). Liver is Wood, Wood

			1	2	3	4	5	6	7	8	9	10
			Wo		F		E		M		Wa	
			Chia +	Yee −	Ping +	Ding −	Wu +	Ji −	Geng +	Shin −	Ren +	Gui −
		Opening Times	GB	Li	SI	Ht	St	Sp	Co	Lu	Bl	Ki
23.00-01.00	Tzu +	↓		SI2		Co3		GB38		St36		
01.00-03.00	Chou −		Li2		Sp3		Ki7		Ht3			
03.00-05.00	Yin +	Bl		St43		Bl60		SI8			Bl67	
05.00-07.00	Mao −	Lu	Ht7		Lu8		Li8			Lu11		
07.00-09.00	Chen +	Co		Co5					Co1		GB43	
09.00-11.00	Si −	Sp	Sp5		Ki10			Sp1		Ki2		
11.00-13.00	Wu +	St		Bl54			St45		Bl66		SI3	
13.00-15.00	Wei −	Ht	Lu5			Ht9		Lu10		Li3		
15.00-17.00	Shen +	SI			SI1		Co2		GB41		St41	
17.00-19.00	Yu −	Li		Li1		Sp2		Ki3		Ht4		
19.00-21.00	Shu +	GB	GB44		St44		Bl65		SI5		Co11	
21.00-23.00	Hai −	Ki		Ht8		Lu9		Li4		Sp9		Ki1

Table 14.

generates Fire, and the Fire point of Heart is Ht8. It opens at the Yin Branch following Yee-Yu, which is Yee-Hai. This is followed by the Earth point of Spleen, Sp3, opening at the next Yin period, Ping-Chou, and the Metal point of Lung, Lu8, at Ping-Mao, and the Water point of Kidney, Ki10, at Ping-Si.

Following on with the Stems, we next come to Ping or the Small Intestine, opening at the Yang Branch *preceeding* the previous example, which is Shen. Therefore SI1 opens at Ping-Shen, followed by St44 at Ping-Shu, Co3 at Ding-Tzu, Bl60 at Ding-Yin and GB34 at Ding-Chen.

This approach provides what one might term the philosophy behind the succession. An alternative way is simply to take the Stems in order and apply, successively, the Tsing, Yong, Yu, Ching, Ho points of the concerned meridians. The results are the same.

For the sake of convenience, the successive opening points are:

GB44, SI2, St43, Co5, Bl54,
Li1, Ht8, Sp3, Lu8, Ki10,
SI1, St44, Co3, Bl60, GB34,
Ht9, Sp2, Lu9, Ki7, Li8,
St45, Co2, Bl65, GB38, SI8,
Sp1, Lu10, Ki3, Li4, Ht3,
Co1, Bl66, GB41, SI5, St36,
Lu11, Ki2, Li3, Ht4, Sp9,
Bl67, GB43, SI3, St41, Co11,
Ki1, Li2, Ht7, Sp5, Lu5.

A still further alternative is to make use of the combination table of 60-days, here recapitulated for ease of reference:

1. Chia-Tzu	11. Chia-Shu	21. Chia-Shen	31. Chia-Wu	41. Chia-Chen	51. Chia-Yin
2. Yee-Chu	12. Yee-Hai	22. Yee-Yu	32. Yee-Wei	42. Yee-Si	52. Yee-Mao
3. Ping-Yin	13. Ping-Tzu	23. Ping-Shu	33. Ping-Shen	43. Ping-Wu	53. Ping-Chen
4. Ding-Mao	14. Ding-Chou	24. Ding-Hai	34. Ding-Yu	44. Ding-Wei	54. Ding-Si
5. Wu-Chen	15. Wu-Yin	25. Wu-Tzu	35. Wu-Shu	45. Wu-Shen	55. Wu-Wu
6. Ji-Si	16. Ji-Mao	26. Ji-Chou	36. Ji-Hai	46. Ji-Yu	56. Ji-Wei
7. Geng-Wu	17. Geng-Chen	27. Geng-Yin	37. Geng-Tzu	47. Geng-Shu	57. Geng-Shen
8. Shin-Wei	18. Shin-Si	28. Shin-Mao	38. Shin-Chou	48. Shin-Hai	58. Shin-Yu
9. Ren-Shen	19. Ren-Wu	29. Ren-Chen	39. Ren-Yin	49. Ren-Tzu	59. Ren-Shu
10. Gui-Yu	20. Gui-Wei	30. Gui-Si	40. Gui-Mao	50. Gui-Chou	60. Gui-Hai

Table 15.

If we refer back to our GB opening, this was Chia-Shu, and in the 60-day cycle we see that this is the eleventh period. According to Chinese numerology all odd numbers are Yang and all even numbers are Yin, so the next Yang period would be number 13, or Ping-Tzu. The Stem Ping is Small Intestines, so the next point to open would be on the Small Intestine meridian, and would open at a Tzu time. The next Yang number is 15, or Wu-Yin, thus the Stem is Stomach opening at the Yin period. The actual points concerned would follow the Tsing, Yong, Yu sequence as described previously, and the fourth point would be number 17, Geng-Chen, or the Ching point of Colon, Co5, opening at Chen time, 7-9am, followed by 19, Ren-Wu, or Bl54 opening at 11.00-13.00 hours.

Following Gall Bladder, the Liver opens at Yee-Yu, which is number 22. The next Yin stem is number 24 — Ding-Hai, therefore the Yang point of Heart, Ht8, opens at 21.00-23.00 hours, and so on.

It will be noted that this method will tell us the stem involved and the actual opening time of the point, but will *not* tell us the day of treatment — i.e., in the previous example of Ding-Hai, the Stem Ding tells us it is a Heart point, the Branch Hai tells us it is the Hai period, but it does not tell us that the treatment is administered on a Yee day — only the first approach will tell us this.

The actual opening times of the meridians may be tabulated as follows:

Tzu	(Yang)	
Chou	(Yin)	
Yin	(Yang)	Bl
Mao	(Yin)	Lu
Chen	(Yang)	Co
Si	(Yin)	Sp
Wu	(Yang)	St
Wei	(Yin)	Ht
Shen	(Yang)	SI
Yu	(Yin)	Li
Shu	(Yang)	GB
Hai	(Yin)	Ki

The discerning reader will have noticed that (a) we commenced with the Gall Bladder at Shu time, and (b) the Kidney appears at Hai, with nothing opening on the periods Tzu and Chou. This is because Hai is the beginning of the Yin Branches and the Kidney is the all-important mother of the ancestral energy. The kinetic energy slumbers whilst Yin is at its peak, and awakens in the Bladder 'with the opening of the eyes' at 3am (as in the circulation in the Tendino-Muscular meridians).

We have still to account for the HC and TH meridians and these, as overall aspects rather than Tsang and Fu organs, obey rules of their own. The next Yang or Yin period following the last point of a particular 'organ day' is known as the 'recurring point', and by an 'organ day' we mean the day pertaining to a specific organ.

The last point of an organ day is the last point used with that particular meridian — with the Gall Bladder it was Bl54, which was the period Yee-Wu, and the recurring point is the next Yang period, which is Yee-Shen. With a Liver organ day the last point is Ki10 (Ping-Si) and the recurring point is the next Yin period, Ping-Wei.

These are the opening times of the two meridians with which we are concerned — the recurring point of the first Yang stem — Gall Bladder — for the Three Heaters, and that of the first Yin stem — Liver — for the Heart Constrictor.

However, we do *not* start with the Tsing point. The points are again referred to the 5-Phases, and in a Yang meridian we use the point which *feeds* the organ. We started with Gall Bladder, which is Wood; Wood is fed by Water, therefore we use the Water point. As we are at the moment concerned with the Three Heaters, this is TH2. The opening time is the recurring point referred to above, Yee-Shen, therefore the Three Heater meridian opens with TH2 at the Yee-Shen period.

We then, as previously, proceed to the next Yang Stem — Ping, or Small Intestines. These are Fire, which is fed by Wood, and the Wood point of TH is TH3. The last point of the Small Intestines organ day was GB34 at Ding-Chen, therefore the recurring point is Ding-Wu. TH3 opens at Ding-Wu. Similarly, the next Yang Stem is Stomach, fed by Fire. The Fire point of TH (TH6) opens at the recurring point of Stomach, which is Ji-Chen, whilst TH10 opens at Shin-Yin. The cycle is completed by ending with the Tsing point (Metal is fed by Earth), and TH1 opens at Gui-Tzu.

The Heart Constrictor meridian obeys nearly similar rules, but here we are concerned with the Yin aspect and we use the point *fed by* the organ. Thus with Liver, which is Wood, Wood feeds Fire, therefore we use the Fire point of Heart Constrictor, HC8, which would open as we saw previously at the recurring point of Liver, Ping-Wei. Carrying on, the next Yin meridian is Heart — Fire. Fire feeds Earth, therefore we place the Earth point of Heart Constrictor, HC7, at the recurring point of the Heart organ day — Wu-Si.

The whole process is not quite so complicated as it first appears and for the sake of completion I am now repeating the previous chart of opening times to include the TH and HC meridians. Also included, in italics, are the opening times of the Yuan or Source points. (See *Table 16* overleaf.)

This last group, the Yuan or Source points, open at the *same time* as the *corresponding* Yu point of the 'organ day'. That is to say, with reference to the Gall Bladder, the *corresponding* Yu point is St43 (the third point to open on the GB day) at Yee-Yin, therefore the Yuan point of GB (GB40) opens at the same time, Yee-Yin. Where Small Intestines is concerned, the corresponding Yu point is Co3 at Ding-Tzu, therefore SI4 (Yuan point of SI) opens at Ding-Tzu. Although, in a Yin meridian, the Yu and Yuan points are the same, the Yuan points *as such* obey the above rules, thus with the Liver meridian Li3 as a Yuan point opens at the same time as its corresponding Yu point, Sp3, at Ping-Chou, as well as at its Yu point time of Shin-Wei.

It will frequently happen that there are no points open at the specific time at which the practitioner desires to treat the patient. In this case, tradition avers that the days bear a Yin/Yang relationship to each other, i.e., days 1 and 6, 2 and 7, 3 and 8, 4 and 9, and 5 and 10, and it will be found that points open at that time on the coupled day may be used instead. For example, if one wished to treat a patient on day Chia, time Yin, when no points are listed, the coupled day with Chia (1) is Ji (6), so we could therefore substitute Ji-Yin and use point SI8. Similarly, if we wished to treat on a Shin day we could use points open on a Ping day, because 8 and 3 are in a Yin/Yang relationship. Note that this relationship does not refer to a meridial relationship as in the Tsang/Fu, but purely to the fact that odd numbered days are Yang and the even numbered ones Yin. The theory is based solely upon Chinese numerology.

A still broader method of the Tzu Wu Liu Chu states that all the 'command' points of any meridian are open at any appropriate time during the day of that meridian, e.g., Chia is the Gall Bladder

			1	2	3	4	5	6	7	8	9	10
			Wo		F		E		M		Wa	
			Chia +	Yee −	Ping +	Ding −	Wu +	Ji −	Geng +	Shin −	Ren +	Gui −
		Opening Times	GB	Li	SI	Ht	St	Sp	Co	Lu	Bl	Ki
23.00-01.00	Tzu +	↓		SI2		*SI4* Co3		GB38		St36		TH1
01.00-03.00	Chou −		Li2		*Li3* Sp3		Ki7		Ht3		HC3	
03.00-05.00	Yin +	Bl		*GB40* St43		Bl60		SI8		TH10	Bl67	
05.00-07.00	Mao −	Lu	*HC7,Ki3* Ht7		Lu8		Li8		HC5	Lu11		
07.00-09.00	Chen +	Co		Co5		GB34		TH6	Co1		GB43	
09.00-11.00	Si −	Sp	Sp5		Ki10		HC7	Sp1		Ki2		
11.00-13.00	Wu +	St		Bl54		TH3	St45		Bl66		*Bl64,TH4* SI3	
13.00-15.00	Wei −	Ht	Lu5		HC8	Ht9		Lu10		*Lu9* Li3		(Sp5)
15.00-17.00	Shen +	SI		TH2	SI1		Co2		*Co4* GB41		St41	
17.00-19.00	Yu −	Li	HC9	Li1		Sp2		*Sp3* Ki3		Ht4		(Lu5)
19.00-21.00	Shu +	GB	GB44		St44		*St42* Bl65		SI5		Co11	
21.00-23.00	Hai −	Ki		Ht8		*Ht7* Lu9		Li4		Sp9		Ki1

Table 16.

day, and any of the command points of the Gall Bladder meridian are open at any *Yang* period during that day, i.e., Chia-Tzu, Chia-Yin, Chia-Chen, Chia-Wu, Chia-Shen, or Chia-Shu. Similarly, Shin is the Lung day, and any of the command points on the Lung meridian are open at any *Yin* period (Shin-Chou, Shin-Mao, etc.) of that day.

The times when the various command points are 'open' are:

Point	Time	Point	Time	Point	Time
Lu11	— Shin-Mao	Ht9	— Ding-Wei	HC9	— Chia-Yu
Lü10	— Ji-Wei	Ht8	— Yee-Hai	HC8	— Ping-Wei
Lu9	— Ding-Hai; Shin-Wei	Ht7	— Chia-Mao; Ding-Hai	HC7	— Wu-Si; Chia-Mao
Lu8	— Ping-Mao	Ht4	— Shin-Yu	HC5	— Geng-Mao
Lu5	— Chia-Wei	Ht3	— Geng-Chou	HC3	— Ren-Chou
Co1	— Geng-Chen	SI1	— Ping-Shen	TH1	— Gui-Tzu
Co2	— Wo-Shen	SI2	— Yee-Tzu	TH2	— Yee-Shen
Co3	— Ding-Tzu	SI3	— Ren-Wu	TH3	— Ding-Wu
Co4	— Geng-Shen	SI4	— Ding-Tzu	TH4	— Ren-Wu
Co5	— Yee-Chen	SI5	— Geng-Shu	TH6	— Ji-Chen
Co11	— Ren-Shu	SI8	— Ji-Yin	TH10	— Shin-Yin
St45	— Wo-Wu	Bl67	— Ren-Yin	GB44	— Chia-Shu
St44	— Ping-Shu	Bl66	— Geng-Wu	GB43	— Ren-Chen
St43	— Yee-Yin	Bl65	— Wu-Shu	GB41	— Geng-Shen
St42	— Wu-Shu	Bl64	— Ren-Wu	GB40	— Yee-Yin
St41	— Ren-Shen	Bl60	— Ding-Yin	GB38	— Ji-Tzu
St36	— Shin-Tzu	Bl54	— Yee-Wu	GB34	— Ding-Chen
Sp1	— Ji-Si	Ki1	— Gui-Hai	Li1	— Yee-Yu
Sp2	— Ding-Yu	Ki2	— Shin-Si	Li2	— Chia-Chou
Sp3	— Ping-Chou; Ji-Yu	Ki3	— Ji-Yu; Chia-Mao	Li3	— Shin-Wei; Ping-Chou
Sp5	— Chia-Si	Ki7	— Wu-Chou	Li4	— Ji-Hai
Sp9	— Shin-Hai	Ki10	— Ping-Si	Li8	— Wu-Mao

Table 17.

6.
'WHAT CHINESE DAY IS IT?'

There remains one question which the frustrated reader will still need answering! We have gone on at great length about Chia, Yee, Ping, Ding, Wu days, but how does he know what these are in relation to the normal calendar when he wishes to treat a patient on 4 April?

Fortunately there is a formula which has been devised, from which the correspondencies can be worked out:

(a) Each year is given a 'root number' for the Stem and Branch of that year. This number increases by a factor of 5 for each year except for the year *following* a Leap Year, when 6 is added. (When the cycle of 60 years is completed it recommences.)

1981	1982	1983	1984	1985	1986	1987	1988	1989	1990	1991
15	20	25	30	36	41	46	51	57	2	7
			Leap Year				Leap Year			

(b) Each month is also given a root number, as follows:

Month	1	2	3	4	5	6	7	8	9	10	11	12
Normal Year	0	31	59	30	0	31	1	32	3	33	4	34
Leap Year	0	31	0	31	1	32	2	33	4	34	5	35

(The reader will see that this is obtained simply by adding on the days of the preceding month of the year and deducting 60 whenever the 60-day cycle is completed.)

The formula is simply to add the root number of the year to the root number of the month, plus the number of the day of the month, e.g., 14 March, 1984 is:

1984	March	14th	
30 +	0	+ 14	= 44. Number 44 on our chart of the 60-day cycle is Ding-Wei.

Or, 27 November, 1986 is:

1986	November	27th	
41 +	4	+ 27	= 72 (less 60) = 12 = Yee-Hai.

The duplex Stem-Branch will actually give us the specific year in the 60-year cycle; the name of the Stem alone will tell us which day it is in the 10-day cycle.

Alternatively, provided one knows the number for 1 January in each year, one can simply work out 60-day cycles from this on the calendar, e.g., 1 January 1984 is a Chia-Wu day, number 31. Therefore 14 March would be 73 days later, equals 13 days later less the first 60-day cycle — 31 + 13 = 44 = Ding-Wei day.

1 January 1986 is Yee-Si = 42. 27 November is 330 days later. 42 + 330 = 372, which is 6 × 60-day cycles with 12 days left. Number 12 is a Yee-Hai day.

As I have said, given the name (or number) of the 1 January each year, it is very easy and the work of only a few minutes to mark out the year's calendar in the 60-day cycles in advance.

The appropriate dates for 1984 to 2004 are as follows:

Leap Year	1984	January 1 is	Chia-Wu (31)
	1985	,,	Geng-Tzu (37)
	1986	,,	Yee-Si (42)
	1987	,,	Geng-Shu (47)
Leap Year	1988	,,	Yee-Mao (52)
	1989	,,	Shin-Yu (58)
	1990	,,	Ping-Yin (3)
	1991	,,	Shin-Wei (8)
Leap Year	1992	,,	Ping-Tzu (13)
	1993	,,	Ren-Wu (19)
	1994	,,	Ding-Hai (24)
	1995	,,	Ren-Shen (29)

Leap Year 1996	,,	Ding-Yu (34)
1997	,,	Gui-Mao (40)
1998	,,	Wo-Shen (45)
1999	,,	Gui-Chou (50)
Leap Year 2000	,,	Wu-Wu (55)
2001	,,	Chia-Tzu (1)
2002	,,	Ji-Si (6)
2003	,,	Chia-Shu (11)
2004	,,	Ji-Mao (16)

The perceptive reader will already have noticed, after perusing the above Stem/Branch numbers, that they progress in the same manner as the 'root numbers' given for the years in the first formula given, but are greater by a factor of 1.

7.
ASTROLOGICAL CONSIDERATIONS

The approaches as outlined are, of course, only a part of a more intricate whole. To arrive at a true understanding of the effect of external energies upon the individual we need to know quite a lot more about the individual himself, for his innate strengths and weaknesses will determine the strength and degree of his reaction. These innate weaknesses or otherwise can to some extent be ascertained by a study of his own astrological make-up, and in ancient China the casting of a complete horoscope would be considered essential before attempting any form of treatment.

This would be based upon the cycles of energy appertaining at the time and place of birth, the governing influences in descending order of importance being:

1. Element of year of birth (Stem)
2. Element of animal sign (Branch)
3. Element of hour of birth
4. Element of month of birth
5. Element of country of birth

As we have seen in Chapter 3, each year of the 60-year cycle comes under the rulership of both a stem and a branch — the branch gives the governing 'animal' of the year, the stem the 5-element component. The branches rotate in a 12-yearly cycle, and the person born during each of those years will be presupposed to possess the basic personality characteristics assigned to that particular animal and also the associated 5-Element component governing that branch in that year (see later).

	Years								
Rat	1900	1912	1924	1936	1948	1960	1972	1984	1996
Ox	1901	1913	1925	1937	1949	1961	1973	1985	1997
Tiger	1902	1914	1926	1938	1950	1962	1974	1986	1998
Hare	1903	1915	1927	1939	1951	1963	1975	1987	1999
Dragon	1904	1916	1928	1940	1952	1964	1976	1988	2000
Snake	1905	1917	1929	1941	1953	1965	1977	1989	2001
Horse	1906	1918	1930	1942	1954	1966	1978	1990	2002
Sheep	1907	1919	1931	1943	1955	1967	1979	1991	2003
Monkey	1908	1920	1932	1944	1956	1968	1980	1992	2004
Rooster	1909	1921	1933	1945	1957	1969	1981	1993	2005
Dog	1910	1922	1934	1946	1958	1970	1982	1994	2006
Pig	1911	1923	1935	1947	1959	1971	1983	1995	2007

In so far as personal relationships are concerned, there are certain harmonious and inharmonious combinations:

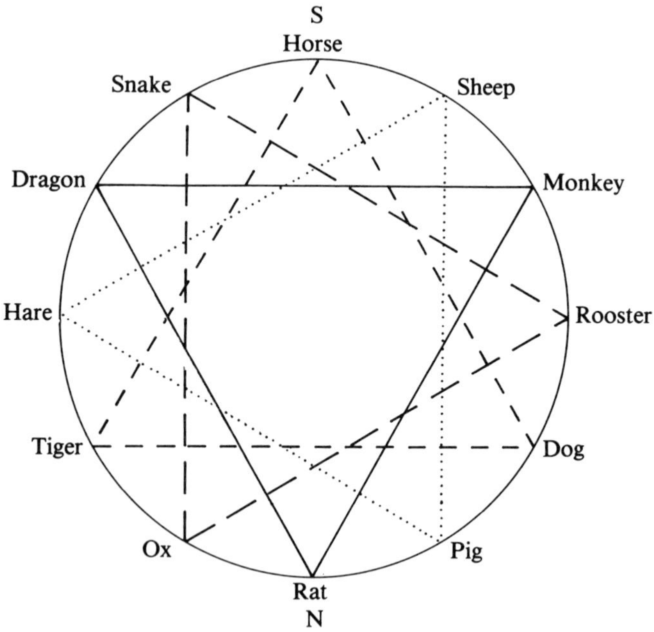

Affinity Triangles

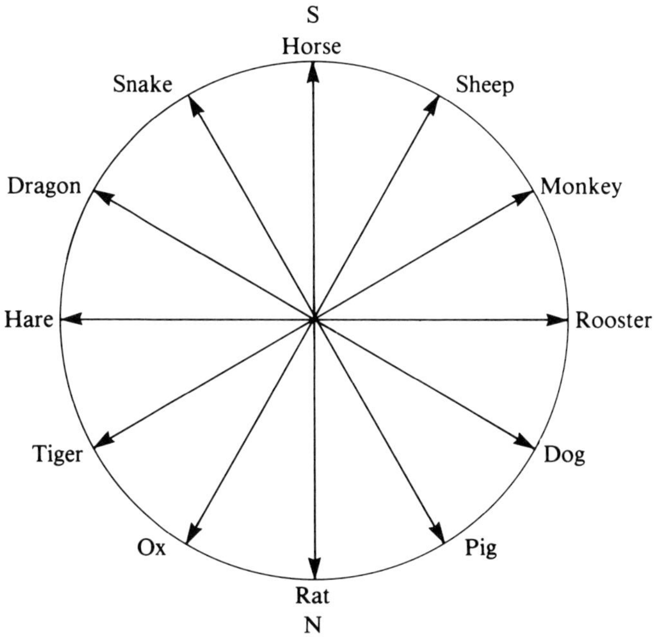

Incompatability

The triad of Horse, Tiger and Dog are the 'sociable' signs. They usually seek to serve humanity, are out-going, impulsive and idealistic. The Sheep, Hare and Pig are artistic types, guided by their emotions. They rely on others for leadership, but can tune-in to their environment and are flexible in their approach. The Monkey, Dragon and Rat are the restless ones; always positive doers who initiate action, they are ambitious and can be short-tempered on occasion. The final trio, the Rooster, Snake and Ox, are the thinkers and planners who pursue their aims with steady determination.

Where the corresponding element of the year is concerned, we must *not* use the correspondencies given in Table 8 — these were the seasonal influences of the Chiaos based on the 24 divisions of the year. The elements of the year used in astrology start off with the familiar 5-Element pattern and, starting with 1984, as that was the first year of the new 60-year cycle, are:

Rat	February 2, 1984 to February 19, 1985	Wood (+)
Ox	February 20, 1985 to February 8, 1986	Wood (−)
Tiger	February 9, 1986 to January 28, 1987	Fire (+)
Hare	January 29, 1987 to February 16, 1988	Fire (−)
Dragon	February 17, 1988 to February 5, 1989	Earth (+)
Snake	February 6, 1989 to January 26, 1990	Earth (−)
Horse	January 27, 1990 to February 14, 1991	Metal (+)
Sheep	February 15, 1991 to February 3, 1992	Metal (−)
Monkey	February 4, 1992 to January 22, 1993	Water (+)
Rooster	January 23, 1993 to February 9, 1994	Water (−)
Dog	February 10, 1994 to January 30, 1995	Wood (+)
Pig	January 31, 1995 to February 18, 1996	Wood (−)

It will be seen that as we have a 12-year cycle and only ten elemental influences, in the next 12-year cycle commencing 1996 the Rat will be Fire+ and so on, each new 12-year cycle commencing with the next 5-Element phase to the preceding one. In 1965 Dragon was Wood+; in the next year of the Dragon, 1977, it was Fire+. In 1989, Dragon is Earth+, so some calculation is necessary to estimate the exact influences at work.

As in all previous instances, the Branches are modified by the Stems, and we can thus have a person born in an Earth Rat year, a Wooden Snake year, etc. The element of the stems will be constant, but the element of the branches will vary as we have seen, and upon the interplay between the two will depend on the strength or otherwise of the various organs subtended.

The influence of the season of birth is the familiar one:

Date:

Summer
(Summer Solstice to
Autumn Equinox)
June 21-September 23
FIRE

Spring
(Vernal Equinox to
Summer Solstice)
March 21-June 21
WOOD

Autumn
(Autumnal Equinox to
Winter Solstice)
September 23-December 23
METAL

Winter
(Winter Solstice to
Vernal Equinox)
December 23-March 21
WATER

To be considered in conjunction with this is the actual hour of birth where we are concerned with the normal 24-hour cycle of energy flow:

Time:

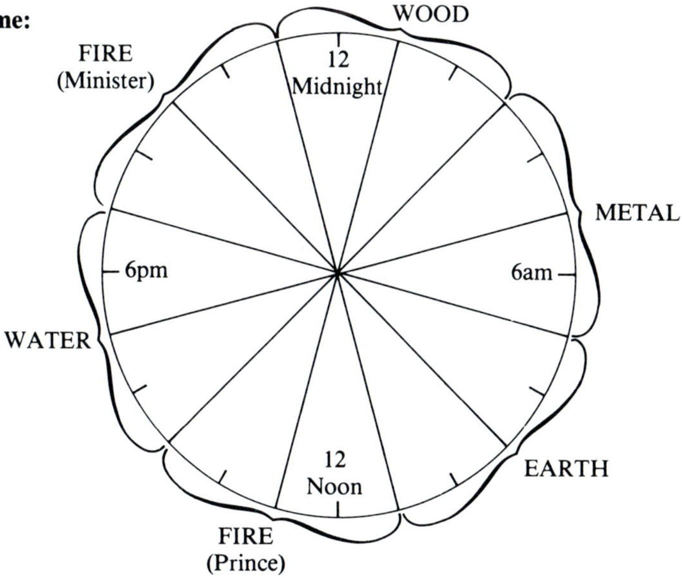

The principal influences of the season and time of birth and the secondary influences of their opposites should be taken into account in each case. As an example, a birth date and time of November 8 at 5.10pm would give a seasonal influence of Metal and a time influence of Water, their opposites being Wood and Metal respectively. In this case, the principal influence would be Metal, with influences also on Wood and Water. The associated functions should show that the patient exhibits strengths or weaknesses of these three elements.

Wood	**Fire**	**Earth**	**Metal**	**Water**
Liver	Heart	Spleen	Lungs	Kidneys
Gall Bladder	Small Intestines	Stomach	Colon	Bladder
Vision	Speech	Taste	Smell	Hearing
Eyes	Tongue	Mouth	Nose	Ears
Muscles	Blood vessels	Flesh	Skin	Bones
Nails	Colour	Lips	Body hair	Head hair
Tears	Sweat	Saliva	Mucus	Urine
Aggression	Joy	Calmness	Sympathy	Caution
Anger	Over-excitement	Depression	Grief	Fear

Birth at change of time or season might indicate the necessity for consideration of either the following or the preceding element.

8.
THE PA KUA AND NUMEROLOGY

'Medicine is so subtle that no one seems able to know about its complete secrets. The way of medicine is so wide that its scope is as immeasurable as the Heaven and the Earth, and its depth is as immeasurable as the four seas . . .'

— *Su Wen*, Chapter 78

So far we have dealt at length with the astrological aspects of the Chinese philosophy. In an earlier chapter we referred to the fact that 'odd' days were considered Yang and 'even' days Yin, and that they bore a Yin/Yang relationship to each other. This axiom

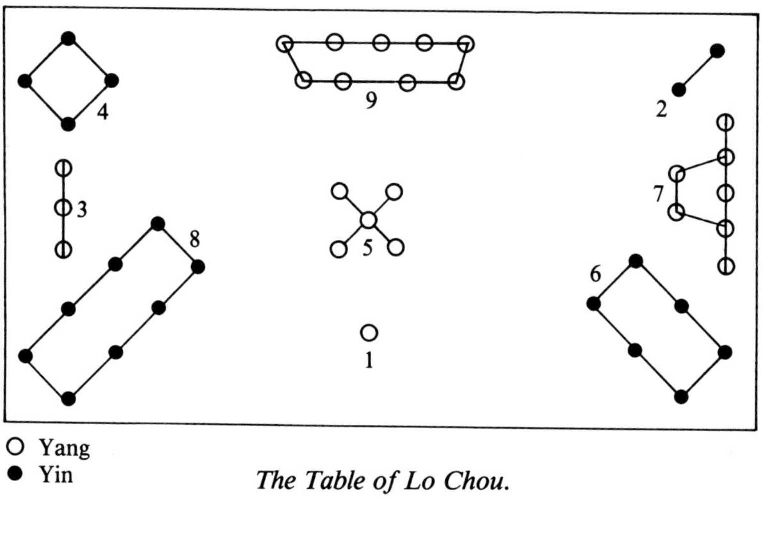

O Yang
● Yin

The Table of Lo Chou.

stems from the fact that inherent in the Chinese astrological approach was their interest in numerology, and an ancient legend refers to the Emperor Yu (founder of the Hsia dynasty, 2205 BC) who one day, on the banks of the river Lo, came upon a giant tortoise on whose shell were inscribed magic diagrams showing the numerological aspects of the creation, from 1 to 9. These diagrams were called 'The Nine Palaces', or the 'Table of Lo Chou'. (See diagram on page 75.)

Before we proceed any further, let us briefly consider the well-known hexagrams of the *I Ching*. These, astrologically, showed the progression of energies through the celestial vault, symbolized by dividing the Heavens and the Earth into eight demi-palaces.

The supreme Yang, shown by an unbroken line ——, was placed in the South.

Yin, demonstrated by a broken line – –, was placed in the North.

East and West are shown by a combination of these two traits, the underlying one representing the dominant energy and the one above it that energy which is beginning to change, thus:

East is ⚎ (Yang energy predominating, with the Yin energy of winter changing into Yang)

South is ⚌ (Pure Yang)

West is ⚍ (The Yang is fading, and Yin begins to predominate)

North is ⚏ (Pure Yin)

In the eight trigrams of Fou Hi, the Pa Kua, corresponding to the eight branches of the 'Rose of the Winds', we find this concept developed into greater detail. Starting with the North, the preparation for spring in the NE shows the Yang base which is beginning to rule but two Yin ☳ traits showing the strength of the still present Yin energy. The East has the basic Yang influence with growing Yang on top and a medium Yin ☲. The SE shows the growing basic influence of Yang, with a final departing Yin

☱ influence. The South is strong, full Yang ☰. In the SW, the Yin energy is creeping in underneath but Yang is still strong ☴, although the — — underneath shows that Yin is predominant.

The West shows two traits of Yin with a medium Yang ☵.

The NW shows the two Yin traits, and a final departing Yang ☶.

North shows the pure Yin of the winter solstice, ☷.

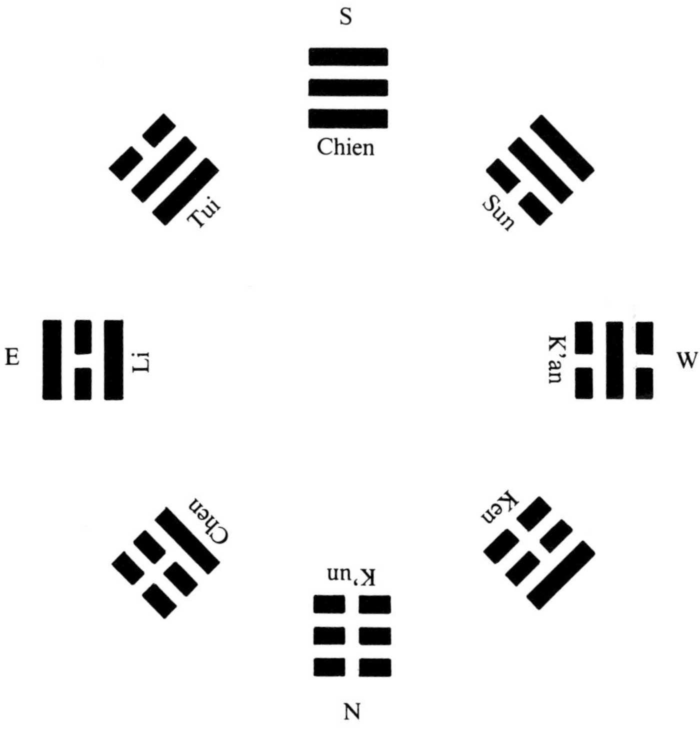

'Former Heaven'.

The Pa Kua as shown is sometimes known as the 'Former Heaven' sequence, as it is the classical description of the formation of the energies and their basic evolution on a celestial level, but it will be noticed that it differs radically from the table of Lo Chou given earlier. This, translated into terms of trigrams, gives what is known as the 'Later Heaven' sequence:

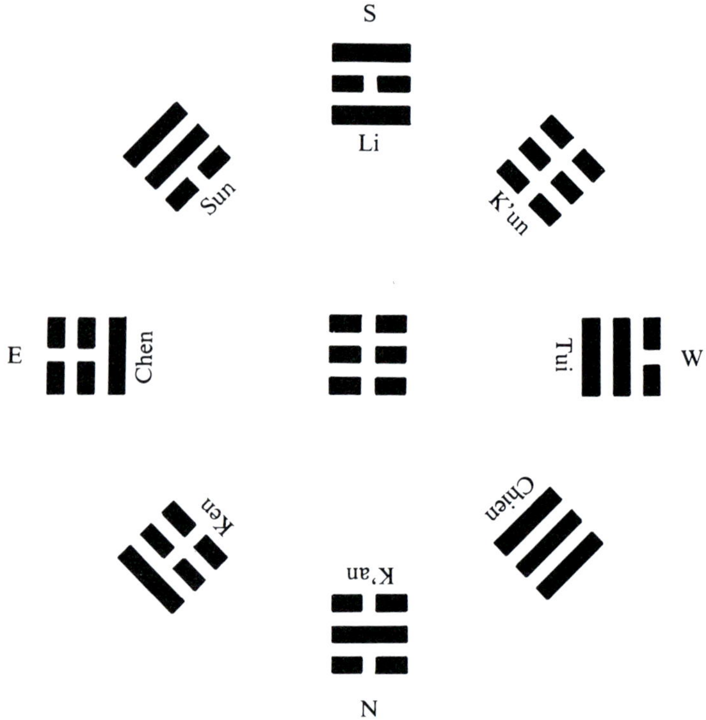

'Later Heaven'.

which is also equated with a 'magic square' which fits in with the Lo Chou table:

4	9	2
3	5	7
8	1	6

In this the numbers in every line, whether taken horizontally, vertically or diagonally, all add up to 15. This is the number of days in each of the twenty-four divisions of the solar year, whilst if we take the opposing Yang and Yin numbers we find they all add up to 10:

9 + 1 Yang = 10 — Old Yang (extreme positivity)
2 + 8 Yin = 10 — Young Yin (slight negativity)
3 + 7 Yang = 10 — Young Yang (slight positivity)
4 + 6 Yin = 10 — Old Yin (extreme negativity)

15 = 10 + 5, which is the Celestial number plus the number of the central energy of Earth.

It must be understood that the 'Former Heaven' Pa Kua represent the energies of Heaven — the table of Lo Chou and the 'Later Heaven' Pa Kua represent the creative energies of Heaven made manifest, and in this classification both the Winter Solstice (1) and the Summer Solstice (9) are Yang, because they are uneven numbers. 1 corresponds to the original Unknowable, the Supreme Unity, from which Yin and Yang emerge; 9 represents the cosmic energy of the Heavens as manifest on the Earth ('Heaven has the

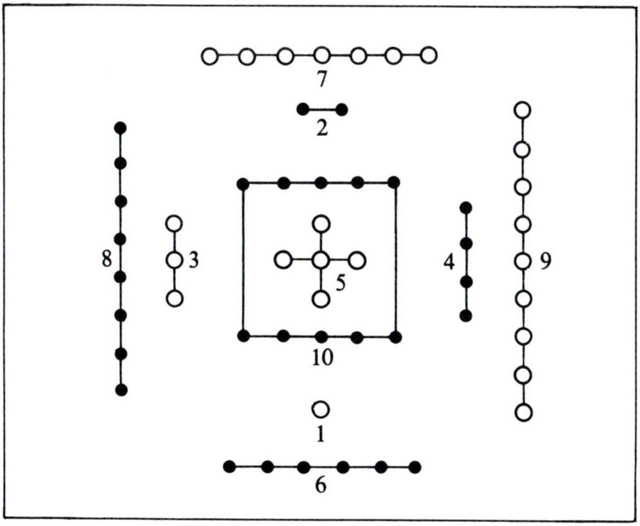

The Table of Ho Thu.

Laws, Earth has the Rules') — the Nine Rules governing the terrestrial energy, the Nine Kingdoms, the Nine Types of Needle, etc.

It was on the banks of the river Lo that a giant tortoise presented the Emperor Yu with the Lo Chou table or diagram. On another occasion he encountered a dragon-horse on the banks of the Yellow River, and inscribed on its flanks was what has come to be called the Table of Ho Thu (see diagram on page 79) which also has a form of 'magic square' associated with it:

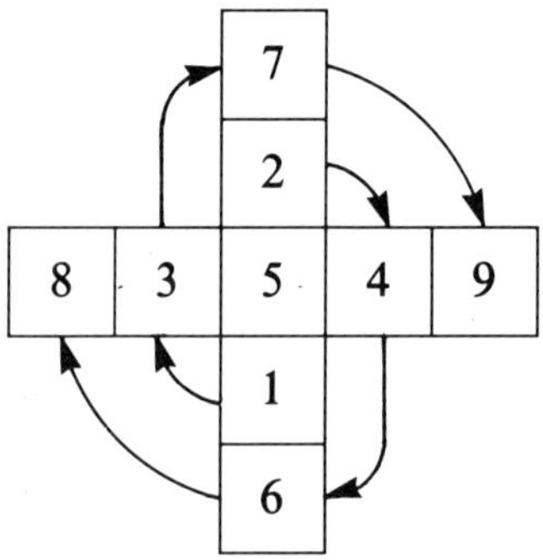

This is one of the earliest approximations to the swastika form in Chinese symbolism, and its actual significance is that it incorporates the numbers appropriate to the Five Elements, Four Seasons, etc. in their correct symbolical connotations and, disregarding the central 5 and 10, both even and odd numbered groups add up to 20.

As the Table of Lo Chou represents the manifest energy of Heaven upon Earth, and is circumscribed by the number 9, so that of Ho Thu represents the Celestial energies, those of the 'Former Heaven', and is circumscribed by the number 10.

Numerically, 1 = Water and the North
2 = Fire and the South
3 = Wood and the East
4 = Metal and the West
5 = Earth and the Centre

The numbers 1-5 are emblematic of generation and are the strongest, numbers 1, 2, 3 and 4 standing for Celestial Energy manifest on Earth, the effect of cosmic energies on the four divisions of space. 5 is the central pivot; creative energy leaves it and returns after spreading to the four quarters. It is the image of the Tao and the uniter of the Tao energy. The remaining six numbers bring in the seasonal correspondences:

6 = 5 + 1, i.e., 1 = Water and North, 6 = season of Winter
7 = 5 + 2, 2 = Fire and South, 7 = Summer
8 = 5 + 3, 3 = Wood and East, 8 = Spring
9 = 5 + 4, 4 = Metal and West, 9 = Autumn
10 = 5 + 5, — Creation and end of Earth, beginning and end of the seasons.

As a point of interest, it must be stated that according to Joseph Needham the critic Hu Wei showed that the ancient mathematical magic squares of Ho Thu and Lo Chou had nothing to do with the *I Ching* but had been attached to it by the Wu Tai Taoist, Chen Thuan, in the seventeenth century AD.

The Ling Kwei Pa Fa Method

With this brief introduction to Chinese numerology we come to another method of acupuncture known as the Ling Kwei Pa Fa, or 'The Eight Techniques of the Spiritual Tortoise' — referring to the legend mentioned earlier about the way in which the Table of Lo Chou was discovered.

If we look at this table, according to the sixth century commentator Chen Luan it is possible to transpose the position of the numbers to the corresponding positions on the human body:

		9		
	4		2	
3		5		7
	8		6	
		1		

Where 9 is on the top, 1 is at the bottom, 3 is on the left, 7 is on the right, 4 and 2 are the shoulders, 8 and 6 are the feet, whilst 5 is in the centre.

Each of these numbers is under the control of one of the Eight-Extra meridians:

1 = Yang Chiao, control point Bl62
2 = Yin Chiao, ,, Ki6
3 = Yang Wei, ,, TH5
4 = Dai Mo, ,, GB41
5 = Yin Chiao, ,, Ki6
6 = Chong Mo, ,, Sp4
7 = Du Mo, ,, SI3
8 = Yin Wei, ,, HC6
9 = Ren Mo, ,, Lu7

or

Ren Mo

Dai Mao   Yin Chiao

Yang Wei   Yin Chiao   Du Mo

Yin Wei   Chong Mo

Yang Chiao

This raises numerous queries but, for the sake of clarity, I will detail the method as outlined first, and attempt to deal with one or two questions later.

To use this method one needs two further small tables, one representing the Stems and Branches on a 60-day cycle and one giving them on a periodic or 60-hourly cycle. (These tables are taken from Dr Henry Lu's *Time-Honoured Chinese Techniques of Acupuncture*):

Stem	Chia, Ji	Yee, Geng	Ding, Ren	Wu, Ping Gui, Shen
Branch	Chen, Shu, Chou, Wei	Shen, Yu	Yin, Mao	Si, Hai, Wu, Tzu
Number	10	9	8	7

60-day Cycle.

Stem	Chia Ji	Yee Geng	Ping Shen	Ding Ren	Wu Gui	
Branch	Tzu Wu	Chou Wei	Yin Shen	Mao Yu	Chen Shu	Si Hai
Number	9	8	7	6	5	4

60-hourly Cycle.

It will be seen from these tables that each Stem or Branch has a specific number assigned to it, and the next step is to work out a calculation based on a formula:

$$\left(\frac{\text{60-day cycle}}{\text{Stem no. + Branch no.}}\right)+\left(\frac{\text{Hourly cycle}}{\text{Stem no. + Branch no.}}\right)\div \text{by either 9 or 6}$$

The remainder is the number required. Division by 9 or 6 depends upon whether the day is Yang or Yin. 9 is a Yang number, 6 is Yin — on a Yang day (i.e., Chia, Ping, Wu, Geng, Ren) divide by 9; on a Yin day (i.e., Yee, Ding, Ji, Shen, Gui) divide by 6.

As an example, on a Ping-Shu day at a Yee-Yu period:

$$\begin{pmatrix}\text{Ping} & \text{Shu}\\ 7 + & 10\end{pmatrix} + \begin{pmatrix}\text{Yee} & \text{Yu}\\ 8 + & 6\end{pmatrix} = 31 \div 9 \text{ (Ping is Yang)} = 3 \text{ with a remainder of } 4.$$

Therefore 4 is the number needed, and from our list we see that number 4 is Dai Mo = GB41, so this is the point we will select for use.

There are also one or two other methods based on similar principles, but their use is all rather specious.

Of all the many queries to spring to mind, the first must of necessity be the relationship of the points used with regard to the numbers. The eight trigrams have their traditional relationships with the Six Chiaos, and these in their turn are related to six of the Irregular Vessels (the other two are obvious):

Ken ☶ — Tai Yin — Dai Mo
K'an ☵ — Chueh Yin — Yin Wei
Sun ☴ — Shao Yin — Yin Chiao
Chen ☳ — Tai Yang — Chong Mo
Li ☲ — Yang Ming — Yang Chiao
Tui ☱ — Shao Yang — Yang Wei
Chien ☰ — Du Mo
K'un ☷ — Ren Mo

If we use the Lo Chou ('Later Heaven') Pa Kua, and substitute the above relationships of the trigrams, we arrive at a very different picture:

Yang Chiao

Yin Chiao Ren Mo

Chong Mo Ren Mo Yang Wei

Dai Mo Du Mo

Yin Wei

From the point of view of control by the Irregular Vessels over different parts of the body, this looks like a slight improvement over the original proposition but I still do not find it very convincing.

The next step would be to see how it would look if we applied the same approach to the 'Former Heaven' sequence, and this gives us a picture of:

Du Mo

Yang Wei Yin Chiao

Yang Chiao Yin Wei

Chong Mo Dai Mo

Ren Mo

This definitely looks a little more promising — at least we've got the Yang up the top where it belongs, but it is possible that with this line of thinking we are branching far away from the original concept of a specific point being influenced at a specific time and day, and are attempting to combine what are actually, not incompatible, but simply parallel, lines of thought. And a definition of parallel lines is that they never meet.

9.
TREATMENT BY THE SEASON

There is one final use of points according to season which, although not actually part of the Stems and Branches concept, is worth including for the sake of completion.

If we remember our seasonal cycle of energy, it can be drawn as:

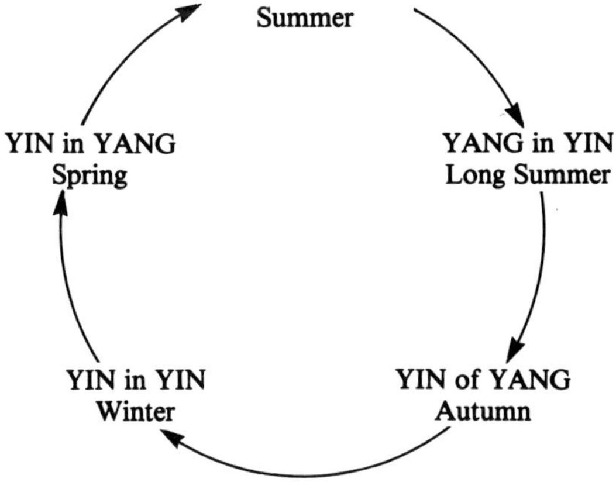

We now need to recollect our cycles through the antique points, and also the entry of energy up the meridian from the Tsing point (these examples are with acknowledgements to Drs Chamfrault and Van Nghi):

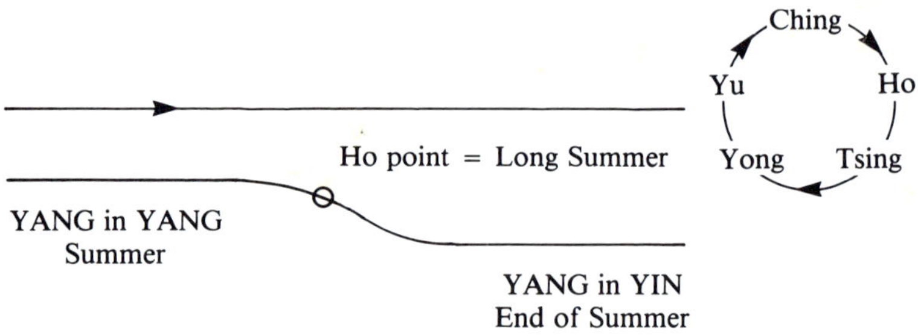

Yang Meridian.

In a Shou Yang meridian the energy starts in the most Yang (superficial) zone and carries on up the meridian to go deep at the Ho point, where it becomes Yang in Yin (Yang energy in a Yin zone). As Yang in Yin corresponds to long summer, so the Ho point also corresponds to long summer and therefore, following the Sheng cycle, the Tsing point must correspond to autumn. This is why, in a Yang meridian, the Tsing point is the autumn (or Metal) point.

(In a Tsu Yang line, the energy emerges from the Ho point (Yang in Yin) and proceeds to the Tsing point via the Yang in Yang — becoming less Yang as it progresses to the Tsing point, and this is understandable because the feet are in contact with the Yin of the earth itself.)

In a Tsu Yin (leg) meridian, the energy ascends from the Tsing point, where it is Yin energy in a superficial zone, i.e., Yin in Yang, and goes deep at the Ho point to become Yin in Yin:

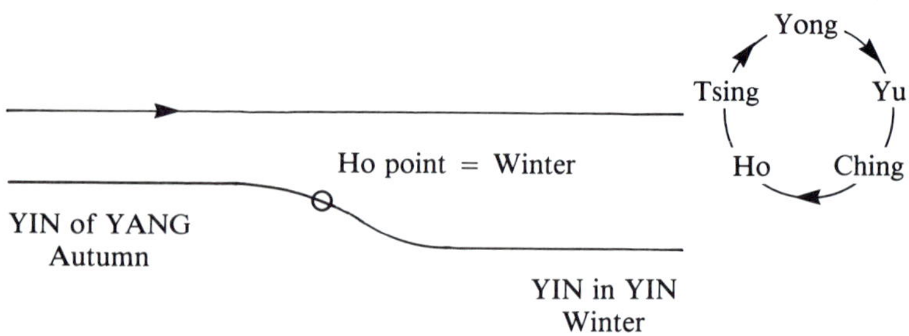

Yin Meridian.

As the Ho point is Winter, the Tsing point must be spring, or the Wood point.

In the Shou Yin line, the energy emerges from the Ho point and descends from Ho to Tsing, with its maximum Yang at the Yong point.

An increase in energy in a meridian can come only from its coupled meridian, from the Tsing point upwards. It reaches its climax at the Yong point and then decreases to, as we have seen, go deep at the Ho point. That is to say, in a Yin meridian we have *Yang* energy entering in from its coupled meridian (e.g., St/Sp), and in a Yang meridian Yin energy enters, to gradually decrease as it partakes more and more of its host meridial energy.

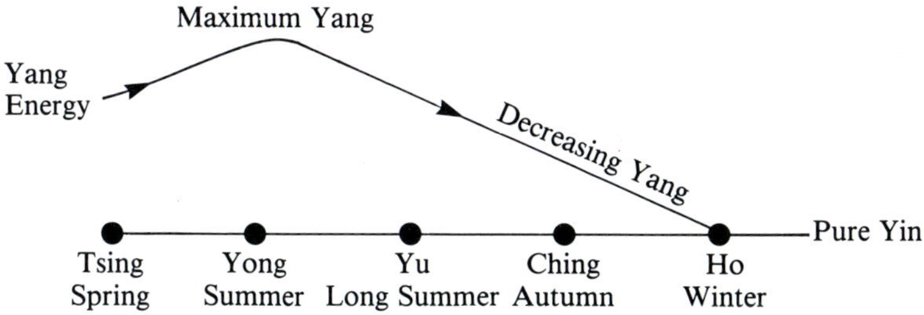

Tsu Yin Line.

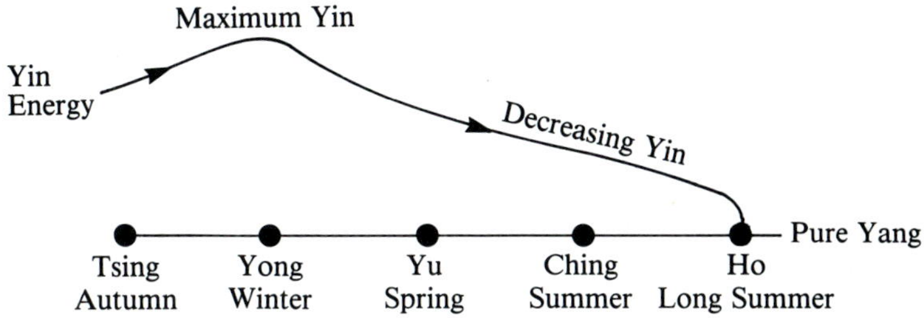

Shou Yang Line.

Every practitioner will remember the basic rules of treatment:

When an organ is empty, to tonify it we follow the energy to reinforce it.

When an organ is full, to empty it we go to meet the perverse energy to disperse it.

This, we can see, is the same as the Mother/Son law. To tonify an organ we use the point of the season preceding the one in which treatment is taking place, i.e., in a Yin meridian, if it is in the Winter we would tonify the autumn (i.e., Ching) point; if it is spring we would tonify the winter (i.e., Ho) point. In a Yang meridian, to tonify in winter we would use the autumn, i.e., Tsing, point, whilst in spring we would use the winter or Yong point.

To disperse an organ we 'drain the Son' — i.e., the points of the following season. To drain Yin, in winter we use the spring — Tsing — point, in summer the long summer or Yu point. In a Yang meridian, in spring we disperse the summer or Ching point, in winter the spring or Yu point.

It is easy to work these out for oneself, but they can be equally easily tabulated:

		Season in which used				
		Spring	*Summer*	*Long Summer*	*Autumn*	*Winter*
To Tonify:	*Yin*	Ho	Tsing	Yong	Yu	Ching
	Yang	Yong	Yu	Ching	Ho	Tsing
To Disperse:	*Yin*	Yong	Yu	Ching	Ho	Tsing
	Yang	Ching	Ho	Tsing	Yong	Yu

* * *

This approach has sometimes been given by authors as a 'Celestial Stems' method. As we have seen, it really has nothing whatsoever to do with them, but is an interesting — if rather specious! — approach nevertheless.

(There is another alternative explanation as to why a Yin meridian has its Tsing point in Wood whilst a Yang meridian begins in Metal: The Yin energy follows a yearly cycle which starts in spring, or Wood; the Yang energy follows a 24-hour cycle which starts at 3am in the Lungs, or Metal . . .!)

* * *

The Yellow Emperor said:

> What a shining way and what a bright theory. Please let me record them on the jade plate to be stored in the golden book-case entitled, Heavenly Energies Circulation.
>
> — *Su Wen*, Chapter 66.

BIBLIOGRAPHY

Allen, Grant, *The Evolution of the Idea of God* (Watts & Co., 1931).

Chaumfrault, A., *De L'Astronomie à la Medicine* (Editions Coquemard — Angouleme, 1963).

Chaumfrault, A. & Nguyen Van Nghi, *L'Energetiques Humaine en Medecine Chinoise* (Imprimerie de la Charante, Angouleme, 1975).

Fortune, Dion, *The Mystical Qabalah* (Williams & Norgate, 1935).

Frazer, Sir J. G., *The Golden Bough* (Macmillan & Co., 1914).

I Ching, Richard Wilhelm trans. (Routledge & Kegan Paul, 1951).

Jeans, Sir James, *The Mysterious Universe* (Cambridge University Press, 1930).

Jung, C. G., *The Collected works of* (18 volumes) (Routledge & Kegan Paul).

Larousse, *Encyclopedia of Mythology* (Hamlyn Pub. Co., 1959).

Lau, Theodora, *Chinese Horoscopes* (Souvenir Press, 1979).

Lu Gwei-Djen & Needham, J., *Celestial Lancets* (Cambridge University Press, 1980).

Needham, J., *Science and Civilisation in China* (Vols. 2 and 3) (Cambridge University Press, 1962).

Nei Ching (*Su Wen, Ling Shu* and *Nan Ching*) Complete translation by Henry Lu (Academy of Oriental Heritage, Vancouver, B.C.).

Lu, Henry C., *The Time-Honored Chinese Techniques of Acupuncture* (Academy of Oriental Heritage, Vancouver, B.C.).

Porkert, M., *Theoretical Foundations of Chinese Medicine* (M.I.T. Press, Cambridge, Mass., 1974).

Rawson, P. & Legeza, *Tao* (Thames & Hudson, 1973).
Rinpoche, Rechung, *Tibetan Medicine* (Wellcome Institute, 1973).
Sakurazawa, Nyoita, *La Philosophie de la Medecine d'Extreme Orient* (J. Vrin, Paris, 1959).
Skinner, Stephen, *The Living Earth Mantle of Feng Shui* (Routledge & Kegan Paul, 1982).
Tao Teh Ching — Arthur Waley translation (Allen & Unwin, 1934).
Thakkur, Chandrashekhar, *Introduction to Ayurveda* (ASI Pub. Inc., 1974).
Blavatsky, H. P., *The Secret Doctrine* (Theosophical Pub. Co., 1893).
Churchward, J., *The Sacred Symbols of Mu* and *The Lost Continent of Mu* (Ives Washburn, N.Y., 1931).

INDEX